The Natural Way

A Complete Guide for Pregnancy, Birth and Motherhood

Susanne Green

DEDICATION

To my daughters and husband, without whom this book would not have been possible. Thank you for your unwavering support and constant encouragement. I would also like to thank my brother, who provided invaluable encouragement and editing assistance throughout the writing of this book. This book is dedicated to all of you

Contents

ABOUT ME AND INTRODUCTION

I am a mother of two girls born 18 months apart. While I had wanted a non-medicalized birth for both, the lack of preparation and knowledge in delivering a baby naturally resulted in two very different outcomes for my daughters' deliveries. The wisdom and learning experience from my first pregnancy greatly informed my second, and that is why I have decided to write this book: to inform and educate other women who may be in a similar place as I was when I gave birth to my first child.

As a theater nurse who regularly sees cesareans being performed, before I became pregnant, I often thought that if I were ever to become pregnant, it would be through an elective cesarean where you walk in all packed and ready to go. No labor, no pushing or screaming. Everything is calm and everything is in complete control. However, after becoming pregnant, I realized my thinking was skewed by several pre-existing notions of what labor and birth really are. It was like a light switch turning on in my head, and I knew I wanted a completely non-medicalized, natural birth. Suddenly, when I became pregnant, I began to see the cesarean delivery of babies in a different light. I would feel for the mother and baby not being able to hold each other immediately after birth. I would wince at the obstetrician complaining about the "laboring woman upstairs who rejected the 'evil hormones' and should just suck it up and have a cesarean." I decided I wanted nothing to do with this for my own pregnancy.

I felt invincible during my first pregnancy. I figured I would be able to have a natural birth with no preparation. I took no advice; I did little reading and assumed I would have the water birth I imagined. I think this method might actually work for some women, as having confidence in your abilities goes a long way when having a natural birth. However, my first pregnancy I suffered from constant sciatic pain and other common aches and pains. The labor was long and the birth ended with a posterior baby, a forceps delivery, and emergency surgery after the birth of my baby; the highly medicalized birth that I did not want to have.

Learning from my mistakes, my second pregnancy I prepared myself as if I were going to run a marathon. I researched foetal positioning and how it can make or break a natural birth. I took tried and true advice from Nana, who had six children at home in six years, on how to have an easy natural birth. My second pregnancy and birth was the polar opposite to my first. My preparation worked. My pregnancy was comfortable and my labor was easy. My baby was born in the water without any medical intervention, and I was able to be discharged from the birth center four hours after her birth.

The difference in result from my new approach astonished me. I discovered that our modern lifestyles, which are very sedentary compared to past generations, have hindered the natural birthing process. We are so bombarded with negative associations of birth from women who want to share their "horror" stories and prove they went through the worst birth imaginable, and from Hollywood movies showing birth as a medicalized procedure where the woman is screaming her head off, that it fosters a bad mindset towards natural birth. Gone are the days where it was normal to have your baby at home and having the advice of elder women in your family who would be encouraging you during a natural labor.

This book is written with the intention of sharing information that can be beneficial in creating a positive, healthy, and natural pregnancy and birth. It focuses on preparing yourself and your partner mentally, emotionally, and physically. However, it is important to note that this is not a comprehensive guide on what to expect during pregnancy, as every woman, pregnancy, and birth is unique. Women who have had multiple children will tell you that each pregnancy can vary tremendously. The one thing that I can say with certainty that will apply to all women is that your attitude and ability to think positively, even during these new and sometimes rough or unexpected times, will make a world of difference in how you cope and handle your transition into motherhood. This book focuses on preparing your mind and body, while also providing helpful ideas and principles that a first-time mother may not be aware of. In today's society, many young people have moved away from their families, resulting in a loss of valuable education and support that was traditionally passed down from grandmother to mother to granddaughter. With the influence of the internet, social media, and other sources, it is easy for new mothers to feel bombarded and overwhelmed. This book aims to provide a guiding hand for new mothers and to help minimize unnecessary worry or anxiety, so that new mothers can feel confident in their bodies' abilities to birth their babies naturally.

PART I – THE PREPARATION PHASE

The key to a successful, easy, and natural birth is preparation. This section covers everything that a new mother-to-be needs to prepare for, including: preparing her mind, which pertains to her attitudes and expectations about the birth; readying her body, which includes details on her general health, exercise, and how to align her body to promote optimal fetal positioning for a natural birth; and finally, a detailed, minimalist, and natural guide to purchasing for a new baby. It is my hope that through this preparation and hard work, a new mother will be able to smoothly go through labor and delivery and be on her way to becoming a relaxed and calm mother.

Chapter 1: Preparing your Mind for Baby

It can be difficult to comprehend that you are going to have a baby. It might not even sink in that it is going to happen until you are holding your baby in your arms. But that first moment when you hold them and look into their eyes is one of the greatest moments of your life. You feel like you have just accomplished something that no one else has done before, even though countless women have done so before you. The fact is, no one has accomplished what you have just done because your birth was unique and you created a tiny individual who you have the responsibility to love and raise to be a functional member of society. This is the single greatest thing you can do for yourself, your family, and your community.

Preparing mentally for your new baby involves learning to relax and to become accepting of the things that are not in your control. Pregnancy can be a difficult time for some women, especially "A" type personalities who crave constant control in their lives. During pregnancy, it can feel like you have lost control of your body, your mind, your energy, and your ability to work and participate in the things you enjoyed before pregnancy. However, your reaction, attitude, and ability to adapt, be calm, and be positive are completely in your control. This chapter will discuss how you can take control of your mind to have a happy and relaxed pregnancy.

Wiring your Brain for Happiness

"The systematic training of the mind, the cultivation of happiness, the genuine intertransformation by deliberately selecting and focusing on positive mental states and challenging negative mental states is possible because of the very structure and function of the brain. But the wiring in

our brains is not static, not irrevocably fixed. Our brains are also adaptable." - The Dalai Lama

By understanding that our brains are fluid through the practice of simple techniques such as gratitude and positivity, we can take control of our thought processes, emotions, and experiences. In very simple terms, your brain works by neurons, or brain cells, making connections with other neurons in the brain that create pathways that make up your nervous system. Every time you perform an action or think a thought, these connections are solidified, making them habitual. This means that the more you react to a certain situation with a negative emotion, the stronger these neural connections become, and this thought process becomes a habitual reaction. Conversely, the more you react to a situation with a positive attitude, the more your brain will be wired for happiness.

Practicing Gratitude

There is significant evidence that has shown that practicing daily gratitude can wire your brain for positivity and allow a person to handle stressors and adapt to change better than those who do not practice gratitude. Pregnancy and birth will create great changes in your emotional and physical condition, as well as being physiological stressors to your body. Incorporating a daily ritual of practicing gratitude will have you well on your way to wiring your brain for happiness during this impactful stage of your life.

Practicing gratitude can come in many forms: daily journal writing, meditation, or simply taking a few moments each morning when you wake to think of at least three things you are grateful for. This does not mean thinking negatively, such as comparing yourself to the less fortunate, but by being positive and counting your blessings. Even the smallest thoughts of gratitude, such as being thankful for your family living nearby, your healthy baby growing in your womb, your good health, your home, having a favorite café to visit, are enough to start wiring your brain for happiness. For anything that makes you feel happy and gratitude for, concentrate on that thought and observe how it makes you feel. The more things you can find that make you feel grateful, the more your brain will seek out similar positive affirmations, which, over time, creates an overall positive impact on your mental health.

This concept might seem hard to believe for some, but there is scientific evidence supporting the power of gratitude and positivity. The act of being grateful stimulates the production of dopamine, the "happy hormone," which will encourage your brain to seek out more things that you are grateful for. This means that the more you practice gratitude, your brain will be programmed to seek out these positive thoughts, leaving you feeling happy, calm, and ready to handle anything that life throws at you.

Seeking Out Social Contacts and Forming Bonds

Just the simple act of knowing you're not alone and that what you're going through is normal can be enough to make you feel relaxed and happy about pregnancy and birth. This is where pregnancy courses, breastfeeding association classes, pregnancy yoga and meditation sessions, and local pregnancy meetups, walks, or groups can become powerful sources of companionship from those who know what you're going through. It is important to understand that the internet and its various forums and message boards are not the place to find this companionship. They are devoid of true human interaction and can be a breeding ground for misinformation. Women are inherently wired to crave the companionship of other women, and face-to-face social interactions are the best solution. Even if you are busy with work or feeling tired, most women can find at least an hour a week to set aside for these personal interactions.

During these times, it is important to see who in your immediate family and friends you can have for support and to strengthen those pre-existing bonds. For those far from family and support, you should seek out other pregnant women in the neighborhood. It is amazing how the bond of motherhood can be enough to start a conversation and even foster a friendship. Many friendships have been established between pregnant women or between mothers in similar stages of life in the aisles of a grocery store or when walking in the park. If you are unable to go out, make sure to engage in face-to-face video chats over messaging groups or social media to foster a closer and more personal relationship. You should carry on these online relationships in real life where possible. Technology can be a wonderful way to initially connect, but once socialization is available, you must pursue face-to-face friendships for your mental health and well-being.

Depression

Hopefully, these simple steps will be enough for the majority of pregnant women to wire their brains for happiness. Unfortunately, pre- and postnatal depression are serious issues that affect many women and may require more help to find happiness. Depression is nothing to be ashamed of and can be managed with help from your loved ones and your healthcare provider. Hormone imbalances during and after pregnancy are major causes of pre- and postnatal depression, which means that the depression felt is often transient and can be overcome when hormones correct themselves over time. On top of this, the recent pandemic put undue stress and fear in many pregnant women and mothers, leading to more instances of postnatal depression.

Practical Activities for Mental Wellness

To prepare your mind for pregnancy and birth, you must first wire your brain for happiness by following the recommendations outlined in this chapter. Here are some other activities you can incorporate into your daily routine that will further help you feel positive and improve your overall mental health:

- **Get outside and walk every day.** Being outside in fresh air will lift your spirits and make you feel energized. Incorporate a daily ritual of walking. Not only is walking good exercise, but it has been shown to have positive effects on your mood as well as health-boosting properties such as improving blood sugar, reducing the risk of heart disease, and is an easy way to maintain body weight. A daily routine of walking can be continued after you have your baby, which will help you stay positive as well as helping to make your baby calmer and happier. There is also evidence to show that babies who are outside and exposed to fresh air often have a lower risk of developing allergies later in life as they are exposed to pollen and dust in fresh air.

- **Be social with other pregnant women or mothers in your neighborhood.** Create a community with those in the same situation as you for social support. These bonds that you form with your peers in your community will be the foundations for friendships and support as your children grow. Being social and having someone to share both the happy and not-so-happy moments in your life can have a very positive impact on your mental health.

- **Maintain friendships from before your pregnancy through face-to-face or meaningful exchanges such as phone calls, letters, or video calls.** It is important to keep bonds with those who might now be at a different life stage than you. These friendships are important as they will maintain your sense of self after becoming a parent.

- **Focus on your partner and make time for each other.** Working to maintain a positive relationship with your partner will help you stay stable and focused on making a happy family for your child. Simple gestures such as making sure to hug and kiss every day go a long way to making a happy relationship. By strengthening this bond, you will be solidifying the foundations for a strong and happy family.

- **Be kind to yourself.** One way to maintain happiness is to be kind to yourself. Never push yourself past your limits, especially during pregnancy when it is easy to overexert yourself. To prevent burnout, it's important to recognize your limitations and take time for self-care regularly. Make time to schedule regular solitude and do activities that you enjoy, such as reading, swimming, taking a bath, getting a pregnancy massage, painting or drawing, or playing music. Anything that makes you feel relaxed and happy is fair game.

- **Take daily quiet time to rest or meditate.** Taking time to rest and meditate daily can help your brain rest and reset, allowing you to maintain a positive mindset.

The Influence of Social Media on Pregnant Woman

The detrimental influence of social media on the mental health of young women is astounding and needs to be addressed in the context of the rise of postnatal depression. The pressure women face trying to keep up with an unattainable image they see on social media can bleed into their pregnancy and birthing process. Making unrealistic expectations of how your pregnancy and birth should go based on someone you follow on the internet, which could in reality be a completely fabricated narrative, will be detrimental to your mental health and overall well-being. Your pregnancy and birth are going to be unique to you and do not have to conform to any doctrine described by an 'influencer'. It is fine and can be beneficial to watch the process of natural birth while you are pregnant. However, it will be better for your mental health to seek out natural birth documentaries that are geared towards empowering women to have a natural birth. Your midwife or healthcare provider may even be able to supply such videos from women who are willing to share their positive birthing stories and videos.

Not only does unnecessarily comparing and holding yourself to unrealistic standards lead to depression, but using social media as your main source of human interaction and for socializing will never compare to the benefits of face-to-face human contact. Women, especially during pregnancy and birth, need to strengthen intimate relationships with friends and family. It takes a village to raise a family. Practicing digital minimalism and eliminating social media during your pregnancy and beyond will help you strengthen your bonds with real-life people. These strengthened relationships will be invaluable once your baby is born, when you have people who are physically and emotionally there for you to help. You will find out very quickly who your real support network is by eliminating social media. This group will include the people who actively seek you out in person and are there to physically help you during your pregnancy and beyond. Even relationships with family and friends overseas will be heightened by eliminating social media. Use technology with the intention of strengthening bonds with people separated by physical distance. Person-to-person calls or video calls, letters, and emails are far more intimate than pressing a like button or scrolling through pictures online.

Social media is highly addictive and can be toxic when used inappropriately. It is manufactured with the intention to make you addicted by feeding you tiny hits of dopamine. Dopamine is a hormone that activates the reward and pleasure centres of your brain. Every time you get a 'like' or a comment on social media you receive a small hit of dopamine. This becomes highly addictive and is the same strategy that coin slot poker machines use.

Pregnancy can be a good time to scale back or eliminate social media use. This will not isolate you, as relationships that are nurtured through physical contact are far more beneficial than superficial interactions online. You will find your true friends are the ones that still reach out to you beyond social media through phone calls, thoughtful letters, and gatherings. New mothers will find these types of interactions much more fulfilling than scrolling down a phone. It is not about shunning the internet or technology, but about using it tactfully. Online research, video calls, organizing pregnancy classes or meet-ups, are all examples of positive ways to use technology with purpose.

Also, consider reducing your exposure to the media and news while you are pregnant and looking after a newborn in order to keep you in a positive frame of mind. The media typically uses sensationalism and fear tactics to spur viewership, and it can be upsetting for a pregnant woman to hear about devastating news constantly. It is fine to keep up on current events, but sheltering yourself from unwanted stress can be the best thing for a nervous and anxious mother-to-be. Tell your partner or family to keep you updated on any news that is paramount for you to know and stop yourself from being overly fixated on being up to date. "Doom scrolling" is a term that has been coined to describe the downward spiral people get caught in when continually browsing through negative news articles on social media. It is easy to feel like you have blinders on when you are only bombarded with negative stories and can feel like it looks hopeless. It is important to realize that the media never shows the whole truth. Fear and sensational news stories sell. It is best to avoid it so you can keep your positive outlook and provide a calm environment for your baby to grow.

The best way to prevent depression and wire your brain for happiness is to get out in the real world. Go outside, make friends with other pregnant women, go for walks every day, and make special time for you and your partner to bond and become excited for your new baby. Get off the phone and internet and enjoy life. You will find that once you have your baby, you will see everything with fresh, new eyes. Babies are wonderful at reminding you to enjoy the simple things in life: seeing leaves flutter in the trees, watching the wind rustle the grass, or seeing a spider spin its web. These are all little things that we would miss and not gain pleasure from if we had our heads in our phones.

Preparing your Relationship for Change

Spending time and focusing on your relationship with your partner before having a baby is crucial for creating a healthy and happy family. Having a baby can amplify the strengths of a relationship, but it cannot fix underlying issues. During pregnancy is the time to nurture your relationship and spend as much quality time together as possible. This means turning off phones in the evening and truly bonding and enjoying your last quiet moments as a couple.

Pregnancy is a time to let go of past issues and any resentments towards your partner, and focus only on the positives. This is the time to give your all to your partner and build a strong, loving relationship that you can bring your baby into. Communication is key to a healthy relationship during pregnancy and beyond. Start by discussing your hopes and dreams for your family. Make it a positive discussion where you can both get excited to start a family. Discuss your parenting styles and beliefs, and be open to compromise. Remember that parenting styles and beliefs can change once you have a child, so be flexible.

Pregnancy is a time when many women find themselves emotional and easily upset. It is important not to nit-pick your partner during this time and to treat them with respect. This relationship will serve as a model for your children's future relationships, so it is important to set a good example. Try to be kind and understanding towards your partner, and let go of small quirks or habits that might bother you. Focus on the positive traits that made you fall in love with your partner in the first place. The baby should not be the center of your universe; your relationship with your partner should remain the foundation of your family. If the parents are happy, the children will be happy, and the family unit will be strong and healthy.

Remember that your partner is also going through a big transition. While you are going through the physical process of pregnancy, they are also facing a major life change. They may have concerns about supporting the family financially, being a good parent, or the health and safety of you and the baby during the birth. It is important to be understanding and try to see things from their perspective. Men often process and react to change differently than women, so it is important to not assume that their emotions or reactions reflect a lack of excitement or interest. Allow your partner to process things in their own way and try to have an open and understanding approach in your relationship.

"Make it a habit in pregnancy to schedule a weekly date night where you focus entirely on each other. This should be maintained consistently after the birth of your baby. A date night does not necessarily have to mean getting dressed up and going to dinner and a movie. It can be as simple as sharing a small moment of quiet together over a coffee in the backyard or curling up together on the couch with popcorn and a movie in the living room. Once the baby is born, this method of utilizing any small moment you can while the baby sleeps is very effective. If you are constantly seizing these moments of free time to enjoy each other's company, you will find your relationship will prosper. Grab any chance you get to steal a kiss and always hug and kiss and say, 'I love you' when saying goodbye. This type of affection is good for your children to grow up watching, as it will set them up for having positive associations of what genuine love and affection can look like.

Before the birth of your baby, if it is in your means, consider planning for you and your partner to go on a 'baby-moon.' A baby-moon is a term to describe one last holiday as a twosome. You can do this at any time in your pregnancy, but it is a good idea not to travel too far while pregnant, as flying for long hours can be uncomfortable and increase your risk of deep vein thrombosis. There is no need to go to great lengths or travel far away. Even booking a hotel in your town or city can be a fun way to relax and enjoy yourselves. Remember, you are pregnant, so long flights or car rides are not relaxing and put unnecessary stress on your body. Aim for something close and fun. Try viewing your town through the eyes of a tourist and do something fun that you have not tried before."

This is a good time to let your nesting instincts kick in and turn your bedroom into an oasis. Order new bed sheets to give your room a hotel-like feel. Take everything out of your room, including moving the bed, and give it a deep clean. You will be resting with your new baby here and the cleaner and more comfortable it is, the more you will enjoy your quiet rest time with your new baby and partner. By cleaning and adding new bed linen, your room will feel fresh and new. Enjoy this new, relaxing space with your partner and make a baby-moon at home. Light some candles, turn the lights down, and relax. Read books together, talk, watch a comedy or romantic movie, give each other massages, or do anything that will help you bond and relax before your baby arrives. Just because you are stuck at home doesn't mean you cannot have an enjoyable baby-moon.

Preparing For Work While Pregnant and Beyond

The first trimester of pregnancy can be a shock for new mothers, especially if they were previously very active. It is important to accept your limitations and get as much rest as possible. This can be difficult if you have not yet told your colleagues at work about your pregnancy, but it is important not to push yourself and try to prove that you are tough. Instead, take care of yourself and allow yourself to rest as much as you need.

When to Tell Work you are Pregnant

I am of two minds when it comes to telling your employer that you are pregnant. The traditional belief is to wait until you are 12 weeks pregnant or longer, as you have a stronger chance of the pregnancy being viable. However, my thinking is that even if you lose the pregnancy, it will be reflected in your work and it is better to have sympathy and understanding from your employer and colleagues rather than them thinking you are unmotivated and failing in your duties. Most companies are still far behind and offer little, if any, time off when a pregnancy is lost, leaving most women to use up their sick leave. This culture needs to be changed. Being open and vocal about both the negative and positive aspects of pregnancy to your organization will set a positive example for other women and will create understanding that will help foster cultural change that is more supportive of pregnant women who experience loss.

The first trimester is the time when most women experience the most lethargy and require more rest. If you have not told your employer that you are pregnant, you potentially have three months of feeling tired and possibly suffering from morning sickness in silence. No matter how hard you try to hide it, people will know something is not right. It is better to avoid workplace speculation and announce your pregnancy early. Women working in labor-intensive jobs or dangerous jobs will also have to inform their employer earlier to be put on light duties.

Pregnancy and Working a Desk Job

It is important for desk workers to be aware that their job may pose issues for pregnant mothers because they are required to sit at a desk for long hours. This can lead to poor posture, which can be uncomfortable for the mother and affect the position of the baby. To address this, it is recommended that desk workers alternate between standing and sitting throughout the day. One way to do this is to sit backwards on a chair, which helps to keep the mother leaning forward and creates a "hammock" for the baby to lie in. This is why pregnant women who work in fields and labor-intensive jobs are often able to give birth and return to work quickly - the physical activity helps to position the baby for an easier delivery. Alternatively, sitting on an exercise ball can be a better ergonomic option for desk workers than a traditional office chair. It is also important for desk workers to take breaks and get up from their desk to stretch and walk around frequently to improve maternal comfort and support good baby positioning. A timer can be useful to remind you to get up and move every 30 minutes.

A Healthy Attitude towards Work while Pregnant

There is a lot of societal pressure for women to do it all: have a career, raise small children, and maintain a certain appearance that they can market on social media. This pressure has led to a kind of competition with women all over the world who might be showing an idealized version of motherhood that is neither realistic nor attainable for most expecting mothers. Boasting about being back at work the day after having a baby or juggling kids and work while looking like Kim Kardashian should not be something to strive for, as it is neither healthy for you nor your newborn. Instead, it is important for women to be kind to themselves and realize that life is cyclic. There is no reason to have it all, all the time. Your pregnancy and the period while your children are small is such a small fragment of your life. If you push yourself to reach a standard you think you need at the expense of your health or quality time with your baby, you need to reevaluate your priorities. Life is short, so prioritize your health and your children's formative years over work. Other things can be pushed to the back burner for now while you focus on yourself and your family. There will be time at different stages of your life for all of your goals.

If you feel overwhelmed and have the means to do so, make more time for yourself during pregnancy and while caring for small children. While not everyone can stay at home, many can reduce their hours. Talk with your partner and carefully evaluate your finances. Many people live above their means, spending more money on things like a bigger house, a nicer car, and luxurious vacations with every pay increase. Saving money and living below your means will allow you to have more time for your family. Remember, just because you can afford something doesn't mean you need to buy it. Money isn't everything and you'll soon find that once you have children, the things you valued in the past may not be as important to you anymore. Having a child allows you to see and enjoy life through a newborn's eyes, making everything seem new and exciting again. Simple activities like walking in the garden or going for a stroll in the park can be enjoyable and fulfilling. Consider cutting back on things like eating out, buying a new car, or upgrading your phone when your current one works fine. Larger changes like moving to a cheaper home or selling a second car can also make a significant impact. All of these changes can add up and allow you to work less and focus on taking care of yourself and your baby.

In today's society, there is often little choice for women but to go back to work after having a child, as the cost of living and family dynamics often make their salary vital in supporting their family. If you have the option to stay at home and raise your children, you should feel confident in your decision. Being a stay-at-home mother or father can be a polarizing topic, with strong opinions on both sides. It is important to remember that your decision to stay at home is a valid one, and should not be swayed or questioned by anyone else's beliefs or ideas about what a modern mother should be. Staying at home with your child has many benefits for both you and your child. You, as the parent, will have the most incentive to care for and take a genuine interest in your child. No childcare worker, no matter how good, will ever match a parent's commitment and love.

The pandemic has changed the way many people work, with many losing job security and some now working from home. During these tumultuous times, it is important to ask for and accept as much help as you can get. Just because you are working from home does not mean you can also run a household and care for young children at the same time. Women working from home need help caring for young children, as waiting to work until the children are asleep at night is not a healthy option and will lead to sleep deprivation and being spread too thin. This is where grandparents, friends, or even the retired lady down the road can be helpful in caring for your children in your home while you work from home.

Preparing your Mind for Labor and Pain Perception

To prepare your mind for the act of labor, you must begin preparations during pregnancy. Just as you wouldn't enter a marathon without preparation, you should not go into labor without training your mind and body. Labor pain perception is subjective and varies from woman to woman. Pain perception of birth can be shaped by preconceived notions of what to expect during labor. Many women have grown up watching movies and TV shows that depict labor as a screaming woman in agony, rushed down hospital hallways on a gurney. This fear of labor and birth can haunt a woman throughout pregnancy and can lead to a greater pain perception of labor, which can result in medical interventions such as epidurals, pain medication, prolonged labors, and even c-sections. So, how can you rewire your brain to improve your perception of labor and birth, and help you have an easy, natural birth?

To rewire your brain for a natural birth, you can follow these simple principles:

- Watch videos of animals giving birth: This idea might sound odd, but you'll be amazed at how calmly animals birth their babies. They find a warm, dark area and become deeply relaxed, allowing them to birth their babies without showing any outward signs of physical pain. They are simply performing a natural physiological function. You must ingrain in your mind the mantra: "If a cat can do it, so can I!"

- Watch videos of natural, calm births: Seeking out natural birth documentaries will expose you to calm and natural labors. Watch and rewatch these videos and envision yourself giving birth in this manner. The more you believe it as a fact, the more likely it will happen. If you go into birth expecting pain, you will experience pain. If you go in with a vision of a calm, pain-free birth, your brain will be wired to help you achieve this!

- Guided meditation for a natural birth: If it is within your means, find a local pregnancy meditation group or calm birth workshop where you can practice mindful birth. This is a great way to meet other women in the same situation as you. If this is not available to you, there are many free guided meditation videos online that you can watch to help you gain a trance-like state in order to visualize your calm, natural birth. Please see below for a script you can read and visualize while you meditate. You can record this script in your own voice and play it back to yourself over and over during your pregnancy and even during labor.

Sample Meditative Script for Pregnancy and Labor:
My baby is safe inside my womb.
My contractions are strong and are going to help my baby find their way into my arms.
My body is strong and I am made to give birth.
I have the ability to completely relax my body so my baby can easily pass through my birth canal.
I am relaxed, calm, strong and capable.

The Power of Visualisation

There is a large body of scientific evidence supporting the effectiveness of visualization. It is well known that visualizing an action activates the same areas of the brain as physically performing it. Elite athletes often use this technique to achieve their goals. These techniques are all variations that utilize the power of visualization. The first step to having an easier birth is believing that you can do it and visualizing your ideal birth in detail. Keep this visualization fresh in your mind by incorporating it into your daily meditations.

You should prepare your mind for labor through positive visualization. During labor, there are other techniques you can use to improve your perception of pain, but for now let's focus on preparing for labor itself. This preparation during pregnancy is key to a successful labor and birth. It's never too early to start. Daily visualizations and meditations during pregnancy will greatly contribute to achieving the natural, easy birth you desire. Set aside at least 10 minutes every day to meditate on your positive labor and birth. Find a calm, quiet place where you can sit or lie down, with minimal distractions. Turn off your phone and choose a time when you won't be interrupted.

Be highly detailed in your visualizations. Imagine your healthy, calm baby being gently and effectively moved by your contracting uterus through your dilated cervix and down the birth canal into your arms. Visualize feeling calm and in control throughout the birth and being able to relax all of your muscles to allow the baby to be born easily. Imagine seeing your healthy baby for the first time, your partner's face upon seeing the baby, the smell and feel of your newborn. The more details you can imagine in your natural birth visualization, the more neural pathways will be created to train your brain to physically give birth. You can use your own imagination for these daily meditations or find a variety of free guided pregnancy and labor meditations online to help you relax and visualize your natural birth.

Chapter 2: Preparing Your Body for Pregnancy and Birth

In this section, I will explain how to prepare your body for a natural birth. This chapter will cover the steps you need to take to be in top form for a natural and smooth delivery. Just as you would not attempt to run a marathon without proper training, you must also prepare your body for an easy, natural birth. Labor is a test of endurance, and by taking care of your body during pregnancy, you can effectively handle labor and childbirth, making it a rewarding and enjoyable experience. This chapter will include information on nutrition and supplementation, diet, exercise, and fetal positioning. By taking good care of your body during pregnancy, you can not only alleviate or even eliminate the discomforts of pregnancy, but also prepare yourself for an easy birth.

Prenatal Vitamins

It is beneficial to have a good prenatal vitamin during pregnancy as it can help fill any nutritional gaps in an inadequate diet. Even if you have a perfect diet, it can be difficult to maintain proper nutrition during pregnancy. Morning sickness, food aversions, and changes in taste can cause your appetite to diminish, and some women may even lose weight due to morning sickness in the first trimester.

There are many one-a-day vitamins marketed as all-inclusive prenatal vitamins, but taking multiple separate vitamins may provide more holistic coverage that can be tailored with the help of a healthcare professional to suit your individual needs based on a prenatal blood test. Using multiple vitamin sources also allows you to carefully examine the supply chain of the vitamins and ensure you are getting the highest quality supplements you can obtain.

One-a-day vitamins often have a large dose of iron along with calcium. However, calcium can inhibit the absorption of iron, so it is better to have a prenatal multivitamin with calcium and no added iron. You can then supplement with iron as needed after discussing it with your healthcare professional. Some women may require more iron, such as those with bleeding issues during pregnancy, hyperemesis, or iron absorption issues. The second trimester significantly increases a woman's iron needs, as this is when her blood volume begins to increase. This is a good time to increase your iron intake through diet and supplements. It is recommended to take an iron supplement of at least 40mcg or more from the second trimester to maintain iron stores as your blood volume increases. It is important to take iron supplements at least 2 hours away from calcium-rich meals. Some people find it helpful to take iron supplements at night before bed as it can mitigate nausea that some people experience from supplements, and you will sleep through it.

Folate is an essential vitamin that should be taken during pregnancy to prevent many neurological birth defects. Folate can be obtained through diet from foods such as green leafy vegetables, citrus fruit, liver, egg yolks, and legumes, or through supplements. Folic acid is the synthetic supplement found in vitamins. However, not all folic acid supplements are created equally. Both folate and folic acid need to go through a complicated conversion to become their active form: 5-MTHF. This process is too complex to fully discuss here, but the key point is that folic acid metabolism is complicated and may not always be efficiently metabolized in some women. When this occurs, the synthetic folic acid can build up in the bloodstream, leading to health concerns. To avoid this, it is best to avoid folic acid supplements and look for supplements that contain better-absorbed preparations that bypass some of the conversion steps and are more easily converted into their active form, such as calcium folinate (folinic acid) or 5- methyltetrahydrofolate (5-MTHF), also known as levomefolate or methylfolate.

When researching and discussing with your healthcare professional which supplements to take during pregnancy, keep in mind the quality of the individual vitamins and minerals that make up the multivitamin. This is not a comprehensive discussion of prenatal vitamins, but rather a starting point for your own research and to bring to your attention some information you may not have been aware of when choosing your prenatal supplements.

Diet

During these nine months of pregnancy, it's important to invest in your health and give it your all, as you are not just caring for yourself anymore, but nurturing a growing human being inside of you who you have full responsibility for. This means giving them the best start to life possible. It's okay to indulge in a treat every now and then while pregnant, but on the whole, you should aim to eat as wholesomely as possible. If you tend to snack on "junk food," try visualizing that what you put into your mouth is going directly into your baby. This can help you feel accountable for your baby's health and stop any unhealthy eating habits. Eating a nutritious whole food diet during pregnancy will help your baby grow, improve their brain development, and reduce the chances of having a birth defect. It will also help prevent excessive weight gain in pregnant women, which will decrease the chances of gestational diabetes and improve the chances of having an uncomplicated birth.

Eating a whole food diet that limits processed foods is the easiest way to maintain good health. There is no big, complicated secret method to follow - simply avoid food that comes in packages. If something does come in a package, make sure you read the ingredients and know where every ingredient comes from. For example, if the ingredients in pasta are just wheat and water, those are ingredients you can picture in your head. However, if there are any ingredients such as artificial flavors, additives with numbers, high fructose corn syrup, or anything that you do not know what it physically looks like or where it comes from, do not eat it. I know this can mean giving up convenience foods, but you are growing a baby and can do without for nine months and hopefully beyond, as these new healthy habits begin to become habitual. There is no fad food or diet you need while pregnant, nor any special recipes. Cooking from scratch without the use of processed foods will be infinitely more healthy and beneficial for you and your baby than anything you can find in a package or from takeout meals, which are made and sold to create profit, not to provide nutritional value to their consumers.

A candy bar is a very obvious example of a processed food. However, there are many hidden processed foods that we need to be aware of and limit from our diet, especially while pregnant. Some common household processed foods include pasta sauces, breads, condiments, salad dressings, spreads, granola bars, biscuits, chips, and ready-made meals. These are often sources of hidden processed white sugar, salt, and hydrogenated oil. When transitioning to a whole food diet, it's important to start looking at every packaged food product critically.

However, cutting processed food from your diet doesn't have to be an all-or-nothing approach. It would be incredibly hard to completely eliminate all processed foods from your diet. There will be times when you want to eat out with friends, need to grab a quick bite on the road or during your lunch break, and processed food can be an easy option. Eating mostly unprocessed food and indulging occasionally will still be substantially better for your health and the health of your baby than eating processed foods as a regular part of your diet.

There are varying degrees of processed food, from heavily processed foods that contain many chemical additives to minimally processed foods that contain only a few ingredients. It's important to make a health-conscious decision when you do eat processed foods and choose the most minimally processed product. Heavily processed foods are easy to identify because they have a long list of ingredients that include items that you would not recognize as real foods. For example, a popular oatmeal bar may contain almost 50 ingredients, including high fructose corn syrup, calcium disodium edta, polydextrose, sodium alginate, and artificial colors. These ingredients do not occur naturally and should not be consumed. If you wouldn't eat any of these ingredients individually, it's important to question why you should eat them when they are incorporated into a breakfast bar. On the other hand, there are less-processed oatmeal bars on the market with fewer ingredients. For example, this Australian brand of oat bars contains a total of nine ingredients, all of which are recognizable as household foods: muesli blend (72% whole grain oats, 62%; nuts, 9% [almonds, pecans]; seeds, 9% [sunflower seeds, pepitas, sesame seeds]; sunflower oil; oat flour; cinnamon), glucose, and natural vanilla flavor.

This minimally processed oat bar is a more health-conscious choice than the heavily processed oat bar. However, it still contains oil and glucose (sugar), which are heavily processed food items. This means that although this type of processed food is a better choice than the heavily processed bar, it still contains heavily processed ingredients and should be limited to an occasional food. Whatever the product is, always read the ingredients and make an informed choice. I hope this comparison allows you to make a healthier choice between heavily and minimally processed items while shopping. However, another reason to avoid processed foods is the expense. Both heavily and minimally processed foods should still be limited from your diet as they will be more expensive than preparing food using fresh ingredients that you sourced yourself. But as life doesn't always work out perfectly, there will be times when buying pre-packaged processed foods is inevitable, and having the ability to make the less processed choice is beneficial.

Cooking

Learn to enjoy cooking. This will be a good preparatory start for your motherhood, as you will be feeding and nourishing a growing human in just a few months. If you start eating healthy during pregnancy, your child will benefit not only in utero but while growing up by being fed nutritious food. Start making an effort during pregnancy to seek out fresh, spray-free or organic produce, and go to markets. Enjoy finding the freshest food and preparing it simply. Produce that has been grown spray-free or organic, as well as organic, pasture-raised meats and eggs, will taste infinitely better than any factory-farmed or mass-produced food, and they also have a nutritional profile that is far superior. This will mean the food will need less preparation and less sauce and salt, as it already tastes good on its own. Some might question the cost of eating this way. You will be shocked at the price of packaged food once you remove it. This money can then be used to buy higher-quality whole food. It is also a good idea to go to bulk food stores for your dry goods, such as beans, nuts, and seeds, to save money. Cutting out take-away meals also reduces your food bill for the week, leaving budget for wholesome food.

Eating small amounts but often is a good philosophy to follow while pregnant. During the early stages of pregnancy, this is an effective way to stave off morning sickness. Later in the pregnancy, when your baby is physically pushing on your stomach, reducing its size, frequent light grazing becomes essential. Do not worry about maintaining a regular three-meal-a-day schedule and instead focus on eating a variety (depending on what your appetite will allow) of high-quality, whole foods throughout the day. Being prepared and having on hand small snacks such as nuts and seeds, crackers, fruits, energy balls, or smoothies will provide a way to stave off nausea and nourish your baby without having to resort to unhealthy processed snacks. Smoothies are especially beneficial as you can add whatever you like to make it a complete meal. Ingredients such as nuts, seeds, protein powder, green leafy vegetables, and fruit are great ways to make up for any deficiencies in your diet.

Simple snack ideas for a pregnant woman:

- **Dates, apples, celery dipped in almond or nut butter of choice**: This snack is nutritious and will give a pregnant woman much needed energy and protein. Dates will also help to soften the cervix helping it to dilate more readily when it's time to give birth.

- **Avocado on whole meal toast**: Avocados are high in folate and B6 which will help your baby's brain grow.

- **Popcorn popped in coconut oil**: Popping your own popcorn on the stove in some coconut oil makes a delicious crunchy snack. Coconut oil has been said to relieve morning sickness and constipation. As well as that you can use the oil to rub on your belly to prevent stretch marks. Make sure you buy virgin cold-pressed oil.

- **Trail mix:** Mix up your own raw nut and seed mix to snack on during the day. Keeping a little bag of trail mix in your pocket or purse to snack on throughout the day is a good way to stave off morning sickness while nourishing your body and baby with healthy fats and vitamins.

- **Smoothies:** making a simple smoothie with frozen berries, bananas, milk or plant milk and a handful of raw nuts and seeds can be a very quick and easy snack or even a light meal for a pregnant woman. Adding a handful of fresh spinach or avocado can be good way to consume extra greens in your diet.

Exercise

Maintaining your fitness levels during pregnancy will greatly improve the ease of your birth. Fitness during pregnancy does not necessarily have to include working out at a gym. This is not the time to start new exercise routines or take up weightlifting or a spin class if you have never trained or exercised before. Pregnancy is a time to concentrate on fluid body movements that help align and strengthen your body. Yoga, swimming, and walking are all gentle exercises that will be beneficial during pregnancy. If you do nothing else but walk an hour a day and do gentle stretching at home, this will be more than enough to help your pregnancy and birth. If you are already in an exercise class or gym, great, continue training but do so at a reduced capacity that respects your changing body. If you are new to exercise, start by incorporating daily walking and stretching, which will keep your weight healthy and prepare your body for birth.

It is important to note that the body releases a hormone called relaxin during pregnancy that works to stretch the ligaments in the pelvis and helps to soften the cervix in preparation for childbirth. It also relaxes all the other ligaments in the body. This means it is easy to overstretch ligaments and cause harm during pregnancy. If you are engaging in activities like weightlifting, it is important to decrease the amount of weight you are lifting and focus on stability. Studies have shown that pregnant women can safely lift objects weighing around 10-12kg (22-26lbs) all day long, but larger objects weighing 20-25kg (44-55lbs) can only be lifted safely occasionally during the day. This is nature's way of allowing you to carry your baby all day, but only occasionally carry your toddler throughout the day. Based on this information, it is safe to work out in the gym with weights up to 20-25kg (44-55lbs). Always listen to your body and do not push past discomfort while pregnant.

Below is a list of gentle exercises that you can undertake daily to help prepare your body for an easy natural birth:

- **Kegals:** It's important to protect your pelvic floor during pregnancy. By strengthening your pelvic floor, you will be able to support your growing baby and avoid unwanted incontinence that many women face after having children. It's just as important to learn how to relax your pelvic floor, as this is what you'll have to do during labor to help your baby descend through the birth canal. To perform kegals, first lie down or sit in a comfortable position. To make a proper kegal contraction, visualize lifting your pelvic floor. It should feel like an upward movement. It can help to visualize that you have a tail and you're pulling your tail up between your legs. While you're doing your kegal, there should be no tension or contraction in your buttocks, abdomen, or face. It may take a while to master this exercise. If you're struggling to perform kegals, it can help to insert a clean finger into your vagina while contracting your pelvic floor. You should be able to feel your vagina tighten around your finger. It may be very weak at first, but through practice, it will strengthen. Start by doing ten quick pulses and repeat this for three total sets of ten. This type of kegal will be beneficial in preventing incontinence while sneezing or coughing, as it activates fast-twitch muscle fibers. Then, it's important to practice long hold contractions, as this will provide you with the strength to carry your baby. Perform the contraction and try to hold it for a few seconds, gradually building this up until you can hold the kegal for 10 seconds or more. Perform this at least 10 times.

- **Yoga:** Yoga is a wonderful exercise for both the mind and body during pregnancy. It can be as gentle or as active as you are capable of and is beneficial for all fitness levels. Yoga is beneficial for pregnancy as it will relax and stretch your ligaments, which will align the mother for birth and strengthen muscles. Attending classes for pregnant women can be beneficial for forming new friendships and sharing experiences. Online classes with a teacher or finding free videos online to perform the exercises at home can be beneficial as well. Inviting your partner to join you can create a bonding time and keep both of you focused on your baby. At the end of each yoga session, place your hands on your belly and spend a few moments connecting with your baby and visualizing an easy, natural birth.

- **Walking:** If you can only do one exercise during pregnancy, choose walking. Walking at a good continuous pace, rather than dawdling or constantly stopping and starting while out shopping, is the best exercise for pregnancy and birth. Walking strengthens your muscles, improves your heart health, helps your baby get into a good position for birth, burns excess calories, is good for your mental health, and has many other benefits. Aim to walk at least 30 minutes a day. If possible, 60 minutes a day of continuous walking at a good pace is even better. Labor can be long, and by training yourself for endurance and cardiovascular health now, you will greatly increase your chances of an easy, natural birth. If walking outside, always be safe: avoid excessive heat, drink plenty of water, and never push yourself past your limits. If a lockdown has you stuck inside, you can walk up and down stairs, around the perimeter of the house, in the backyard, or wherever you can – just make it work. Put on headphones and listen to your favorite audiobook or call a friend while you walk to keep you motivated and entertained.

- **Swimming:** Swimming is another great exercise for pregnant women. The weightlessness of being in the water takes the weight of the baby off the mother's back. Swimming, like walking, can improve cardiovascular health and strengthen muscles while being gentle on ligaments. Swimming breast stroke is also effective in helping the baby get into a good position. Try to do laps for at least 30 minutes a few times each week. While it is fun to float and relax in the water, it is important to prepare your body for childbirth, so be sure to do continuous exercise for at least half an hour without a break. Swimming can improve your endurance and help you get through a natural birth.

Rest

While maintaining physical activity during pregnancy is important, it is equally important to get high quality rest during pregnancy. Resting on the couch, scrolling through your phone or watching Netflix all day is not true rest. Your mind will still be stimulated and you may feel lethargic and restless. Instead, try finding activities that help you relax, such as taking a bath, sitting or lying in a calm environment, listening to music or guided meditation, sleeping, or simply closing your eyes without screens. This type of rest will give you a sense of peace and quiet that is beneficial for calming your mind and body and preparing for birth. If this is your first pregnancy, take advantage of any opportunities for solitude, as it won't be long until you have a little shadow following you around and demanding all of your free time.

Chapter 3: Baby Positioning

Having your baby lie in an optimal position within you will help facilitate an easy natural birth. There are several positions a baby can lie in. Head down does not necessarily mean the baby is in the best position. As well as being head down, the baby should have their chin tucked and be facing your back by the 32nd to 36th week of pregnancy. The baby can lie in a less than optimal position but still be able to turn during labor and delivered safely. Having your baby lie in the most optimal position will make labor and delivery progress as smoothly as possible. Optimal fetal positioning will create a shorter, easier labor and help baby be delivered safely. Luckily there are several methods that the mother can implement to coax the baby into the best position that will be discussed shortly.

Firstly we will discuss the various positions that babies can lie in:

- Anterior
    - o Left Occiput Anterior position (LOA) is the most optimal positioning. The baby is head down and facing your back meaning they can

easily slide down your birth canal for birth. You will feel baby's kicks on your right upper side. His firm back will be running down your left side.

- Posterior
    - o Posterior baby is also head down; however, they are facing your front meaning their hard skull is pushing on your spine that can cause a long labor and back pain throughout both the pregnancy and labor. These babies can flip or be born posterior. There is a higher incidence of posterior babies being born via ventouse or forceps.

- Breech
    - o Breach position is when the baby's head is up and their bottom is in your pelvis. The breech presentation can be caused by imbalances in the pelvis from several common causes such as single-sided leg or ankle injuries, carrying children on one hip, driving with one-sided pushing of the pedal. To help baby move into an optimal position you must seek the assistance of a professional experienced in helping with breached babies.

- Transverse
    - o Transverse lie is when the baby is lying side-wise across the womb. This is expected before 29 weeks and they should move to head down by 32 weeks.

This is not a comprehensive guide to baby positioning, but an introduction to show you that head down is not enough. The orientation of the baby's head is very important in facilitating an easy birth. Babies can change position during labor, meaning that even a baby in a less than optimal position can still be born naturally, so there is no reason to become obsessive about your baby's position. However, working on your body to stretch ligaments and increase movement and flexibility will give you a greater chance of the baby lying in an optimal LOA position, resulting in an easier, shorter labor. Even if your baby is in a less-than-optimal position, this preparation will create space in the body so the baby can better navigate the birth canal during birth. Practical actions that you can take to achieve this will be discussed below.

It is now common for women to have babies in hospitals, and some require medical intervention such as c-sections. This was not always the case just a few generations ago, when our great grandparents mostly gave birth at home. The difference in society today is that women are no longer toiling in the fields or undertaking daily physical labor that requires them to be on hands and knees, or very active in general. Modern women are sedentary by nature, with many working desk jobs and driving to work. This means modern women have poor posture that can cause the baby to be in a less than optimal position. This mass shift in lifestyles is one theory as to why more women are having difficulty giving birth naturally.

In order to change this trend in modern women, it is important to increase activity and mobility throughout pregnancy, focusing on being on hands and knees as much as possible. This might sound daunting to a pregnant woman who is tired and juggling many things at once, but the benefits of increasing movement and activity will energize you and prevent or alleviate many of the aches and pains experienced by many pregnant women. This builds on daily exercises by focusing on stretches that will open and align your pelvis. Many of these activities can also be useful during active labor.

Methods to Help Baby Move into an Optimal Position for Birth

- **Rebozo:** The rebozo is a long scarf traditionally used in Mexico by midwives to improve outcomes for pregnant and laboring women. It is made of woven cotton or wool. The rebozo can also be used after birth to carry your baby. You can purchase an authentic rebozo online, but if that is not within your means, a single flat bed sheet folded lengthwise in half can make a suitable alternative. The rebozo can be used during pregnancy to help the baby move into an optimal position and also help the mother relax and feel good because it loosens tight ligaments in the hips, back, and uterus and momentarily takes the baby's weight off the mother's spine, relieving back pain. Here are two methods of how to use the rebozo in pregnancy:

- o Method one: Kneel in a comfortable hand and knee position. Place cushions or a folded blanket under your knees for comfort. Take the rebozo and place the middle section of the fabric around your belly like a hammock. Have your partner, or anyone who is willing, stand behind you with their feet on the outside of your knees. The helper will take the ends of the rebozo and lift until your belly is cradled. They should stand with their feet slightly bent and back straight. The partner should ask and confirm if it feels comfortable. The material should be flat and flush to your belly. You should feel the weight of the baby lifted off your back. At this point, the partner will begin a very gentle shifting motion. The fabric should not cause friction on the mother's belly, but gently jiggle the belly from side to side. This should include very short movements where the partner's hands do not move more than 1 to 2 centimeters from their starting position. This can be very tiring for the partner to do, so you can use this technique for as long as your partner is willing and able. This motion will help relax uterine ligaments and gently cradle the baby into an optimal anterior position. This method can be used daily throughout pregnancy and during labor between contractions.

o Method two: This method is affectionately known as 'shaking the apple tree,' as it involves the rebozo being placed over the mother's buttock and being gently shaken to release tension in her lower back. The pregnant woman kneels down on all fours, and the partner kneels behind her. The rebozo is placed over her posterior, and the partner applies gentle downward pressure by holding the sides of the rebozo. Once again, a gentle shifting motion is applied. Using the rebozo with your partner or support person is also a great bonding exercise that can make your partner feel like they are an active participant in your pregnancy.

- **Posture and sitting:** Having good posture while pregnant can help facilitate a natural birth and also prevent or minimize the aches and pains of pregnancy. To maintain proper posture while pregnant, stand straight while walking and keep a neutral spine. Avoid wearing heels as they will misalign your spine and are also unnecessarily uncomfortable. Slouching and leaning back on the couch or in a chair puts the baby in a bad position in your uterus. You want to think of your belly as a hammock cradling your baby. You can achieve this by sitting on a cushion on the floor, cross-legged with your knees below your hips. This will bring your belly slightly forward and align your hips, allowing your baby to sit in the perfect anterior position. Using an exercise ball to sit on is another good alternative to sitting on the couch. If you are sitting for long periods at work, swap your chair for an exercise ball. This will keep you in a much healthier position. Alternatively, sitting backwards on an office chair will keep you leaning forward slightly, making the baby lie in a better position.

- **Hands and Knees:** Make sure to spend time in the hands and knees position every day. This will make your belly act like a hammock and cradle your baby, allowing them to come into an anterior position. You can get into this hands and knees position in a number of situations, such as when watching TV or playing with the dog. Scrubbing the floors will get the baby into the correct position, give you much-needed exercise, and help keep your house clean. If you are struggling to stop using social media, make a deal with yourself to only use it while on hands and knees. This will minimize your use of it while helping to position your baby.

- **Walking:** Walking one hour or more a day will greatly help position your baby well for birth. Walking will lengthen your back and leg muscles, which will help align the spine and pelvis. Don't push yourself past your limits, and work your way up to an hour a day of continuous walking.

- **Forward leaning inversions:** This position was developed by a chiropractor to help untwist ligaments in the lower pelvis and cervix due to poor posture. It also uses gravity to give the baby more space to rotate into a better position by momentarily taking the baby's head off the cervix. Always consult your healthcare provider before performing this pose. It is safe for most women, but should not be performed by women with bleeding issues. The method is as follows:
  - o To perform the inversion make sure you have a stable base such as a couch or stairs.
  - o Using a support person bring your knees to the edge of the stairs or couch.

- o Slowly and carefully lower your hands and then forearms down to the floor while keeping your knees on the couch and your bottom in the air.
- o Let your head hang freely and do not let it rest on the ground.
- o Hold this position for three deep breaths and then come back up.
- o Preform this pose daily at least three times.

If you are undertaking these daily activities and still experiencing various pains, it could be a sign that you have an imbalance of muscles or ligaments in your body. In this case, it may be beneficial to seek help from a professional bodyworker, such as an osteopath, chiropractor, or physiotherapist who specializes in pregnant women for an assessment. Look for professionals with good reviews or recommendations through word of mouth. Many activities we do throughout the day are one-sided, such as carrying a heavy purse, getting out of bed, vacuuming, carrying children, which can easily cause us to become misaligned. This misalignment can cause the mother to experience pain and make for a more difficult labor.

Chapter 4: Preparing for the New Baby

This section will provide the expectant mother with the bare minimum essentials needed for caring for your baby. It is easy to get carried away and buy an abundance of baby paraphernalia before they are born. This is expensive and wasteful as you will soon find newborns require very little: a safe place to sleep, your breast, diapers, and a few swaddles and clothes. This section will give you the minimalist baby essentials to keep you focused on bonding with your baby and prevent clutter from taking over your house and unnecessarily depleting your bank account.

Baby Shower

Baby showers are a good time to be practical. If you are lucky enough for someone to throw you one, don't hesitate to request the gifts you need or, better yet, ask for cash to contribute to the actual items you need. This is especially good if there is a big ticket item you need, like a co-sleeper cot or nursing chair, which can be expensive. If you feel uncomfortable asking people for money or gifts, another effective option is to request no gifts and only accept hand-me-downs as a sustainable option. You might be surprised by the monetary gifts you receive by just requesting 'no gifts.' On top of that, by accepting all the hand-me-downs offered, you might discover things you liked or needed that you didn't know about. This is not the most minimal option, but as they are second-hand, you can examine your baby shower gifts once you're home and donate or pass on the items you don't like, and not feel too guilty about it as they are second-hand. Instead of requesting monetary or material items, a great gift to ask for is the person's help once the baby comes. This help will be invaluable and so beneficial to a new mother.

Here are some ideas of things to request:

- Home cooked meals brought over that can be eaten now or stored in the freezer
- Help with cleaning the house
- Help doing laundry
- Walking the dog/looking after pets
- Holding the baby while you have a much needed bath and rest

You will be surprised by what people offer when you ask. Most people will want to contribute and help you when you have a baby, and by giving them the opportunity, they will be more than willing to help. Many new mothers can feel pressure to show that they are capable and can do it all by them-selves. There is no shame in taking help, and it will make your life much calmer and relaxed, which means you can invest more of your energy into your baby and into your re-covery from birth.

Cloth or Disposable Diapers

For a significant amount of time, your baby will be in dia-pers. Your baby will wear a few thousand diapers before they become toilet-trained. This produces a substantial amount of waste if using disposables and an even more substantial amount of money. Cloth diapers have a larger upfront cost of purchase than disposables but are more cost-effective over your child's diapering years. They will also survive to be used for subsequent children. There is an element of added work using cloth diapers as you have to launder them. However, thankfully we have modern washing machines that do most of the hard work, and it becomes a matter of loading an extra load of laundry every few days and hanging them out in the sun. The money saved on disposable diapers and wipes is a large driving factor for why many families choose to use cloth.

Cloth diapers are also beneficial as they reduce your child's exposure to chemicals in disposable diapers. There are poten-tially harmful chemicals such as dyes, chlorine, phthalates, and fragrances that are sitting directly on your baby's bare skin from using disposables. Unless the diaper brand you are using explicitly says it is free of a certain chemical, it is best to assume that it is there. There are many brands now marketed as chemical-free that have more transparent ingredient lists on their disposable diapers. So if you make the decision to use disposables, choosing a brand that is trying to reduce exposure to chemicals is a good idea. However, these brands are generally more costly, which needs to be factored into your decision-making.

Cloth diapers have come a long way from the cotton towels and rubber pants used by your grandparents. Modern cloth diapers are much more convenient, with an outer waterproof layer made of polyurethane laminate and absorbent liners made of materials such as cotton, hemp, and bamboo. These diapers are durable and long-lasting, so the initial bulk purchase will serve you for all subsequent children. Buying second-hand and using a laundry sanitizer in the wash can be a good option for budget-conscious parents. Alternatively, new diapers can be purchased in bulk bundles to reduce the cost. The number of diapers you need depends on how often you wash them, how many children you have, and their ages. For a newborn, around 30 diapers should be enough if you are washing every two to three days. Washing cloth diapers is not as daunting as it may seem, but it is outside the scope of this book to provide in-depth instructions. There are many detailed guides available online that provide comprehensive directions based on your specific washing machine, detergent, and water type.

- Newborn stool is water soluble and does not need to be washed off before being put into the washing machine.

- Reusable wipes can be made from cheap flannel cut into squares.

- Store used diapers in a dry hamper in the laundry room. You can roll up the diapers to prevent odor.

- Place an open cup of bicarb soda in your laundry room to keep it smelling fresh.

- Preform a rinse and spin on your diapers everynight until you wash them to prevent urine smelling.

- Wash diapers every 2-3 days or so. It is important to have a full load of diapers as the abrasion from the diapers rubbing against eachother in the wash helps to mechanically clean them.

- Preform two washes on diapers. First a short wash followed by a long wash.
- Always use cold water as to not destroy the PUL.
- Never add bleach or vinegar as they can delaminate the water proof layer.
- Hang diapers in the sun to sanitise them and remove any stains.

Dressing Baby

Most mothers love baby clothes. However, there are a few things a new mother might not think of when choosing baby clothes for her first child. It is easy to get excited and buy every cute ensemble, but it is important to take into account functionality and comfort as well. A pair of overalls may be cute, but they can be a hassle to take on and off multiple times on a squirming and crying newborn. The same goes for a cute dress with buttons running down the back. These buttons can become tiny pressure points that will stick into your baby's back and make them uncomfortable. It is also important to consider synthetic materials or scratchy tags and seams when picking baby clothes. There are several factors you should look for:

- **Ease of dressing:** Onsies with zippers down the front are much easier to take on and off, especially in the middle of the night after a blowout, than onsies with buttons or clips. It's even better if the zipper is two-way, as you can change diapers without exposing your baby's chest. Remember that newborns have delicate necks, so onsies that open at the front with a zip are also beneficial because you don't have to pull a neck hole over their heads!
- **Buttons:** Baby clothes often have buttons on the back of shirts and pants. These can create little pressure points for your baby to lie on and will not be comfortable.

- **Fabric choice:** Always choose breathable, natural, and soft fabrics. Babies naturally run hot, and having them in a synthetic outfit will be uncomfortable, hot, and not good for their delicate skin.
- **Price:** It's not just mothers who love baby clothes. Everyone will love gifting you with clothes. It's important not to waste your money on clothes, as you will probably be gifted many, as well as hand-me-downs. Babies do not stay in one size for long, so the mother who buys many might find the baby grows out of them before they even get to wear them! A good method of purchasing baby clothes is to buy second-hand baby clothes bundles online. These often come with many clothes in one or two sizes for a girl or boy. The benefit of this method is that when your baby has grown out of them, you can re-bundle the clothes and sell them online again. This is not only a sustainable option but a frugal one. Second-hand clothing shops are also a good option.
- **Washability:** Cute clothes often mean hand washing only. Make sure you factor this in when choosing clothes. Delicate lace or fabric flowers do not last long in the washing machine.

Please see the end of book for a checklist on minimal baby clothes essentials.

Bathing Baby

You will notice that in my essential baby checklist, I do not include baby baths or toiletries. There is much marketing and effort put into pushing a wide range of cosmetic products for babies, when in reality their delicate skin needs very little attention. When babies are born, they are coated with a white, waxy substance called vernix. Vernix protects the baby's skin while in the uterus and lasts until around 40 weeks. This is why babies born late might not have any vernix and might have flaking dry skin. It is very beneficial to leave the vernix on their skin, as it will absorb into their skin, leaving it soft and protected, as well as having antibacterial properties. Delaying a baby's first bath allows beneficial good bacteria they picked up from the birth canal to colonize on their skin, which will make their skin healthier. I suggest waiting a few days to bathe your baby. This will also help your newborn's temperature control and help you to establish a bond through skin to skin contact and breastfeeding before you bathe them.

When you do have a baby's first bath, you can do it in the comfort of your home. There is no reason to bathe your baby in the hospital or birth center. The less time spent there, the better after birth. At home, you do not need any fancy infant bath or cosmetics. Try hopping in the bath or shower together, and have nice fluffy towels ready and a heated room to dry baby in. Newborns have poor temperature control, meaning they are very sensitive to cold and heat. Water alone is enough to clean baby. Soft washcloths or konjac sponges with water are nice ways to give baby a massage and gently clean the skin. By using water only, you are also retaining the baby's natural scent, which can promote bonding. Also note that it can be important for bonding to not have harsh smells for both baby and mom. So, avoid perfumes and strong smelling toiletries for the first few weeks, so you can bond with baby. Studies have shown that natural baby smell can curb postnatal depression. So, keep that newborn smell by avoiding soaps and scented baby cosmetics and enjoy smelling your newborn for your mental health.

Other popular baby toiletries include nappy creams, powders, and ointments. The best way to prevent nappy rash is to give your baby's genitals a break from being in a damp and hot diaper by providing daily naked time. A good time to do this is during tummy time. Lay a waterproof mat or heavy towel under your baby blanket before placing your naked baby on their tummy. Sometimes rashes are unavoidable. If you see the first signs of redness on your baby's bottom, increase the amount of daily naked time. A natural zinc-based nappy cream can be used once a rash develops, but it is not necessary to use it on a daily basis. When choosing a cream, make sure to pick one that does not contain preservatives or chemicals such as BHA, fragrance, boric acid, parabens, or talc.

The Baby's Sleep Space

Baby sleep seems to be a huge issue in Western culture that mothers are obsessed with. Babies are expected to go from the comfort of the womb to being able to settle themselves and sleep on a hard, stark mattress all by themselves. Co-sleeping or using a co-sleeper cot that attaches to the side of your bed is a great alternative to having your newborn sleep in a different room. Having your baby close means you can monitor your baby more closely and are more likely to hear if the baby needs you. Waking in the night to feed a baby who is co-sleeping and breastfed is a very good way to stave off sleep deprivation. You simply roll over, take the baby out of the co-sleeper cot and nurse them in bed lying down while you're half awake, then place them back in their co-sleeper cot. It gets even easier if you are co-sleeping in the same bed as you will most likely be still attached to the baby and they will begin nursing without waking you up. The hormones released during breastfeeding also help you fall asleep again faster. This is a far more relaxed approach than having to get out of bed, go to another room, sit up in a chair to feed the baby, possibly having to go to the kitchen to prepare a bottle, then transfer them back to the cot asleep or going through the whole settling routine again. The time your child is a baby is a very short moment in time, and you should be enjoying all of it rather than stressing over a doctrine of sleep that you 'must' follow.

The majority of mothers worldwide sleep with their babies, particularly in Asia, Southern Europe, Africa, and Central and South America. It's interesting to note that many parents in Western countries, such as America and Australia, also sleep with their babies, but it is not openly discussed because there has been a push for babies to sleep in cribs to prevent sudden infant death syndrome (SIDS). The rise of SIDS is not due to mothers sleeping with their babies in bed, but rather a combination of factors including sleeping on unsafe sleep surfaces like couches, beanbags, and car seats, and socio-economic factors such as drug abuse, morbid obesity, and smoking. When these factors are taken into account, SIDS is no more prevalent in co-sleeping babies, and in fact, it can even reduce the incidence. Japan, which has one of the highest co-sleeping rates, has seen declining rates of SIDS that continue to fall as maternal smoking decreases to almost zero and rates of exclusive breastfeeding increase. This shows that it is not necessarily co-sleeping that is dangerous, but rather other contributing factors.

Cultural acceptance of co-sleeping also makes it a safer and more relaxed practice. Western mothers who view co-sleeping as a last resort may feel like they are not performing to societal expectations of having their baby sleep independently. On the other hand, accepting co-sleeping as a safe and culturally accepted behavior means mothers feel no sense of defeat and have the bed safely prepared for co-sleeping. Only using co-sleeping as a last resort when putting baby to sleep in their own room fails means the mother may end up sleeping with the baby on an unsafe sleep surface such as a chair, sofa, or bed that is high off the floor.

Tips for safe co-sleeping:

- Sleep in a warm button-up shirt that you can easily nurse in. It will keep your upper body warm, and you don't want to cover the baby with the comforter.
- Smoking, morbid obesity, and sedating drug use do not mix with co-sleeping.

- Have the mattress on the floor or have a side rail on your bed to prevent the baby from falling off.
- Make sure the mattress and bedding are firm and sleep the baby on their back to sleep.
- Do not wrap or swaddle the baby if co-sleeping.

Establishing realistic expectations before the baby's birth can help you manage your perception of sleep deprivation. A mother who is only woken once or twice at night might feel more sleep deprived than a mother who is woken multiple times. This can be due to various factors such as poor health, diet, and recovery time. However, your attitude can go a long way in helping you feel more rested and calm. A mother who has been woken many times and had little overall sleep can think of it in two ways. The first mother wakes up feeling sorry for herself and worries that she has no energy to do anything that day. This feeling of exhaustion will follow her all day as she fails to rest and pushes herself to perform at her pre-child level. The second mother also wakes up tired and wishes she had more sleep. However, she knows that this is only temporary and is grateful to have a healthy baby and many other things to be thankful for. She knows the baby will have their first nap at nine and decides to leave the dishes in the sink, forget about the laundry, and be kind to herself by turning off her phone and sleeping while the baby sleeps. The mess will still be there when she is rested and has the energy to deal with it.

Every baby is unique and will sleep through the night when they are developmentally ready to. There is no one method that is guaranteed to work for every baby when it comes to helping them sleep. It's important not to compare yourself to others and to do what feels right and gets results for your own baby. If that means putting the baby to sleep while nursing in your arms or in a pram, that's completely fine. I believe that babies who co-sleep feel more secure and are better able to transition to sleeping independently in their own rooms and beds, and sleep through the night when they are ready, without experiencing sleep regressions, compared to babies who were sleep trained with controlled crying methods. Newborns cannot be sleep trained because they have to wake up at night due to their small stomachs, which cannot go that long without milk. Sleeping through the night will come with time, so enjoy the newborn stage and do what you need to do to ensure that your family gets a good night's sleep. When your baby is out of the newborn stage, you can reassess sleeping arrangements and explore a method of sleep that works for your family, whether that be continuing co-sleeping or transitioning the baby into their own room.

Preparing for Breastfeeding

For successful breastfeeding, you don't need to purchase anything or prepare beyond attending a breastfeeding class with your partner. My theory is to not purchase any bottles to feed your baby until you absolutely need it. It's possible to go through infancy without ever needing a bottle as the baby or toddler can go straight to drinking from a cup. Maintain a positive attitude that your breasts are all you need to nourish your baby. Having bottles and formula for 'just in case' sets the precedent that they are there and readily available. A decision you make late at night to just give one bottle could potentially undo your breastfeeding relationship. If there comes a time when you have to go back to work and need to express into bottles, wait until that time comes to purchase feeding equipment. Please refer to the breastfeeding chapter for more information on breastfeeding.

There are many breastfeeding pillows, covers, nipple shields, and other products available that can make breastfeeding seem like an expensive endeavor. The fact is breastfeeding is practically free, minus the 500 or so calories of extra food a breastfeeding mother has to consume. All of the breastfeeding paraphernalia is better left unpurchased until you find that you actually need it. If you'd like to be very minimal, you don't need to buy a single thing to breastfeed your baby. However, if you'd like to splurge on one non-essential but comfortable baby item, it would be a high-backed rocking, nursing chair. When breastfeeding, you spend a large amount of time sitting in one position nursing your baby. Having a comfortable chair where you feel relaxed will be very beneficial in forming a positive breastfeeding relationship and allowing you to rest while you nurse. You can always use the couch, bed, or even nurse on the go in the baby carrier. Whatever you choose to nurse regularly, make sure you're comfortable, relaxed, and have access to your water and a snack.

Prams and Babywearing

Prams can range in price from a few thousand dollars at the high end to cheap second-hand options. Many mothers believe that a pram is a status symbol, but newborn babies are instinctually hardwired to want to be constantly in your arms. This stems from caveman days, when if a baby was left on the jungle floor, it could be eaten by a predator. This is why many cultures still carry their babies in some way, as they have to go back to working the fields with baby in tow. My advice is to use a baby wrap during the first three months or longer, and then once they are older, you can put them straight into a standard pram without needing the expensive bassinet attachment. The next time you go to a shopping center, notice how many babies are being carried while the mother pushes around an empty pram! When looking for a pram, look for ones with a good sun visor. Baby skin is very sensitive, and it is worth having a pram that can protect them from the sun on long walks. Second-hand or hand-me-down prams are a good option for money-conscious or sustainability-minded parents.

Babywearing is an excellent way to transport your baby in the first few months and beyond. The first three months are often referred to as the "fourth trimester," during which baby is still adjusting to the outside world. You cannot spoil a baby. The closer you keep them, the calmer they will be, the calmer you will be, and you will be fostering a bond that will help nurture your baby into a confident and happy child.

Babywearing is beneficial for a number of reasons:

- A calmer baby who cries less
- Hands-free and the ability to get housework done or do other tasks
- Prevents flat head syndrome or other cranial deformities. Babies left to lie in baby swings, car seats, or on flat surfaces can develop deformities. Wearing your baby takes the pressure off their skull and allows for proper development
- Allows you to be more in tune with your baby. Mothers who wear their babies are more likely to see hunger signals and react to other needs quicker than mothers who do not wear their baby
- Ability to go out and about with baby sleeping on your chest. Getting grocery shopping done, going to a café with friends is all much easier while babywearing
- No heavy pram to lift in and out of the car

There are many carriers and wraps available to carry your baby. From traditional stretchy wraps where you wrap a long cloth around your body to wear your baby, to highly structured carriers with straps and buckles that allow you to wear your baby in several positions. It is important to note that some baby carriers are not suitable for newborns or may require an insert for newborns. I believe choosing a more traditional style of baby wrap or sling for the newborn stage is the most beneficial for the first few months. Traditional styles put the baby in a more natural position and cradle them to your body in a way that is similar to how a baby monkey hangs from its mother. Structured baby carriers become more useful once the baby becomes larger. By purchasing or making a wrap or sling for the newborn stage, you can see how your baby wearing progresses. You might find that you love it and change to a structured carrier when they are older, or you may find that after the newborn stage, you are finished with baby wearing and the pram is enough.

Below are a few common baby wraps that are suitable for newborns that can be used from the day the baby is born:

- **Stretchy baby wrap:** This is an affordable and effective way to carry your baby. It is a long, stretchy piece of fabric that you wrap around your body, placing the baby inside against your chest. You can take the baby in and out of the wrap without having to rewrap it, making it convenient to use. Some people may feel intimidated by the idea of wrapping the fabric themselves, but with practice it becomes second nature. One benefit of this style is that it is very ergonomic, allowing you to wrap it to fit your and your baby's size perfectly. You will also be completely hands-free while using this wrap. This wrap is suitable for small babies up to around 9 months, at which point they may become too heavy for it. After that, it may be more beneficial to use a different type of baby carrier, such as a sling or structured style carrier.

- **Sling:** This is another affordable option. It consists of a long piece of non-stretch fabric that is worn over one shoulder. This can be used for newborns as well as toddlers, who can be carried on your hip. One drawback of the sling is that it is one-sided, making it difficult for mothers to carry for long periods of time. However, this can be mitigated by alternating the shoulder you hold the sling on.

- **Woven baby wrap:** The woven wrap is similar to the stretchy wrap, but it is made of a non-stretch piece of fabric. To use this wrap, you must hold the baby on your chest and wrap the fabric around both of you. Like the stretchy wrap, it may seem intimidating at first, but with practice it becomes easy. The rebozo, a traditional Mexican shawl, can also be used as a woven baby wrap. One advantage of the woven wrap over the stretchy wrap is that it can be used to carry your baby into the toddler years, either as a sling or on your back. The drawback is that you cannot take the baby in and out of a woven wrap without re-wrapping it, which can be tiresome with a newborn.

Whatever carrier you choose, always follow its safety guidelines. These guidelines may include keeping the baby in an upright position with their airway clear and face uncovered. Babywearing allows you to be more instinctively aware of your baby's needs. Their breathing and other physiological functions will be regulated by being on your chest, making it a safer and more secure place for your baby.

Preparing your Home for Birth

In reality, there is not much you need to do to prepare your home for a newborn. Since they are immobile, there is no need to baby-proof just yet. However, as many pregnant women know, the nesting instinct often kicks in during the third trimester, causing an uncontrollable urge to clean and organize.

If you find yourself feeling this urge, here are some practical cleaning and organizing tips that will not only make your house clean, but also create a comfortable, inviting home for you to rest and bond with your new baby:

- **Create a nest:** As you will be spending a lot of time nursing, it is important for your mental and physical well-being to set up a "nest" in your house. Take time and care to choose a comfortable, quiet nook in your house, and set it up with a comfortable chair or couch, a blanket, a book, water, and a small snack so you can really enjoy the time you spend nursing. Make an effort to create a serene oasis for you to relax and bond with your baby. Add some beautiful artwork or house plants to give you something visually pleasing to look at. Aromatherapy diffusers or candles can add to the overall calm and pleasant atmosphere. The more you love this area, the more you will enjoy nursing and being still and calm during these special moments with your baby.

- **Minimize clutter:** Minimizing your house is not essential, as the baby does not care how organized your house is. However, decluttering your house will make it infinitely easier to maintain and clean after the birth of your child. New mothers soon find that juggling caring for their baby, their family, and themselves while keeping the house tidy can be difficult. I will not go into depth on how to create a minimal house. You can find a wealth of information on the topic at your local library or online. The main premise is to keep only what you value and make sure there is a place for everything and that everything is in its place.

- **Prepare the baby's room:** Whether you have a beautiful baby room set up or the baby will be in your room, make a clean, comfortable place for the baby. Keep it simple - the sleeping area should be free of toys or pillows. Decorations and toys are fine, but they are more for the parents at this point than the newborn.

- **Prepare your fridge and freezer:** Deep clean your fridge and freezer, and fill them with healthy food. Start freezing leftovers or making simple ready-made meals, such as soups or stews, so you can have quick access to food after the birth of your baby, avoiding unhealthy food or takeout.

- **Scrub the floors:** This will not only get your floors clean, but it will also help get your baby in a good position for natural birth. This can also be done during labor!

PART II - LABOR AND BIRTH

This section of the book will detail the process of labor and birth, taking a natural approach, which involves the use of relaxation, meditation, and water to allow the mother to naturally give birth to her baby without the need for medical intervention. The following chapters will also cover how to choose a care provider, where to give birth, how to relax during labor, and how to have a natural delivery of your baby.

Chapter 5: Active Birth

Active birth is an umbrella term that covers both pregnancy and labor. It begins with implementing the methods discussed in the "Preparing Your Body" chapter to bring the baby into the optimal position for birth, and then progresses to activities to undertake during labor and birth. It promotes the use of the mother's own instincts and working with her labor to do what feels right for her. Active birth encourages women to be upright and move through their contractions. Dancing, walking, swaying hips, squatting, and other movements during labor, along with meditative and relaxation techniques, are encouraged to help a woman easily progress through a natural labor and birth.

Film and media often portray birth as involving a woman lying on her back, screaming and in agonizing pain. However, lying on your back is one of the worst positions to give birth in. Not only is it more painful and uncomfortable for most women, but it also constricts the baby's passageway through the birth canal. This position became popular because obstetricians have better access to the laboring woman when she is on her back and her legs are in stirrups. The rise of medicalized births, where epidurals and other pain medications are given, means that women are confined to beds during labor. A drug-free, natural birth allows freedom of movement during labor and the ability to change positions, which greatly enhances a woman's ability to have a natural, intervention-free birth. Preparing your body for birth through your pregnancy, and then being an active participant in labor and instinctively listening to your body, is the major philosophy of the active birth philosophy.

Chapter 6: What is Natural Birth

Natural birth can mean different things to different people. To some, it may mean any vaginal birth, regardless of medication or medical assistance used. To others, it may mean a completely unassisted home birth. Whatever your interpretation, it is important to make sure your expectations and definition align with those of your support people and doctor or midwife. This book takes the view of natural birth as a vaginal birth without pain medication, such as epidurals or opiates, and instead favors the active birth philosophy, which utilizes pain control techniques such as meditation, relaxation, hydrotherapy, and movement.

There are many positive outcomes from having a natural, non-medicated birth. By utilizing the physical and mental preparation and active birth techniques outlined in this book, you will be able to have a calm, natural, and easy birth without the use of epidurals or narcotics, which will also reduce your likelihood of needing a medical intervention.

There are many advantages of a natural birth, which include:

- Reduced incidence of tearing, as the mother can feel the contractions and instinctively push or relax her body through them. With an epidural, the woman cannot feel the contractions, which may lead to an increased risk of tearing if she has to be coached to push.

- Faster recovery time, as you will be able to get up and move soon after the birth and go home as soon as four hours after the birth of your child.

- Freedom to move and change positions during labor as you see fit.

- The opportunity to catch your own baby as it is being born.

- The option of having a water birth.
- Decreased risks associated with medical interventions and epidurals.
- The chance to see what your body is naturally capable of doing without assistance.
- A baby that is more alert and able to nurse sooner after birth.
- A faster labor, as epidurals can slow the labor process.
- Natural birth allows a woman's own hormones to flood her system, which can aid milk production, bonding, and satisfaction with the birth.

Chapter 7: Why Avoid a Medicalized Birth?

This section will discuss several interventions and pain management strategies that are routinely used in a hospital setting. Women are often not given full disclosure regarding the potential side effects or harm that medicalized interventions could cause to them and/or their baby. These pain management methods and interventions are widely used during labor and birth and are often seen as a "gold standard" by hospitals; but women are not always provided with all the information they need to make an informed decision.

Epidurals

Epidurals are a highly effective method of managing pain during childbirth, but they can also significantly alter the natural process of labor and birth. This is because they are often accompanied by a dose of synthetic oxytocin, which can reduce the mother's production of oxytocin and potentially lead to longer labor times and difficulties with breastfeeding and bonding after birth. Oxytocin is a powerful hormone that plays a central role in both brain function and physiological processes.

In a pregnant and laboring woman oxytocin is used to promote and facilitate a healthy natural birth by:

- Creating strong uterine contractions and preventing postpartum blood loss.
- Creates regular contractions
- Helps to reduce stress and facilitate bonding between mother and baby and gives the mother a feeling of love and happiness
- Skin to skin contact after birth creates high concentrations in oxytocin in the mother which helps birth the placenta and initiate bonding and breastfeeding

Synthetic oxytocin cannot cross the blood brain barrier and cannot elicit the same maternal bonding and feelings of love. By reducing your natural production of oxytocin, epidurals, although an effective pain relieve can be detrimental to a mothers natural hormone production that can diminish bonding and breastfeeding with your newborn. As well as this disruption in hormone production epidurals also have several risk that include:

- Increased risk of tearing as the laboring woman has to be coached through contractions as she cannot feel them
- Lowers blood pressure which can reduce blood flow to your baby. This also means the mother will have to have an intravenous drip for fluids.
- Synthetic Pitocin will be administered to woman with an epidural
- Newborn is more likely to develop respiratory distress in the immediate period after birth with mothers who have had an epidural

- Increased risk of medical interventions and caesareans

Epidurals carry a risk, so the mother and baby must be monitored closely. This may involve the use of IV medication, synthetic hormones to induce labor, and fetal heart rate monitors. The mother may also be confined to bed and coached to push the baby out, leading to a higher likelihood of medical interventions. Epidurals have been linked to an increased risk of assisted birth using ventouse or forceps compared to drug-free birth. They can also alter the body's natural chemistry during childbirth, turning the natural event of giving birth into a highly medicalized one.

Induction

The use of induction methods, such as the synthetic oxytocin called 'pitocin', has increased significantly. Many women who are tired of being pregnant may not realize the risks associated with induction and can be easily swayed into having an elected induction. However, inducing labor in an otherwise healthy pregnancy that is progressing normally has been shown to increase the need for medical intervention and the risk of complications, leading to longer hospital stays. Pitocin-induced labor also disrupts the body's natural hormones, similar to epidurals, and does not help with maternal bonding, breastfeeding, or the release of endorphins, which are important for pain management during natural birth. As a result, women who have inductions are often more likely to need an epidural for pain management. Induction may be necessary in certain medical situations, such as when the mother or baby is compromised or the baby has reached 42 weeks of gestation, but it should be avoided whenever possible as an elective procedure.

Active versus Physiological Third Stage

The third stage of labor is the period after the baby is born until the delivery of the placenta. 'Active third stage management' is a standard intervention in many hospitals, which involves injecting an uterotonic medicine like pitocin to constrict the uterus, followed by early clamping of the umbilical cord and controlled cord traction to help remove the placenta. The theory is that this will prevent postpartum hemorrhage in the mother, as the placenta is delivered in half the time of a natural or physiological third stage. However, in an uncomplicated natural birth, early cord clamping and cord traction to expel the placenta can deprive the newborn of a significant amount of blood. As the baby is born, a bolus of blood is transferred from the placenta to the baby, which is used to perfuse the lungs and prepare the baby to take its first breaths. When this blood is taken away by early cord clamping, the lungs become perfused from other organs, putting the baby in a hypovolemic (low blood volume) state. This deprives the baby of oxygen, iron stores, stem cells, and blood volume. As mentioned earlier, synthetic oxytocin can also negatively impact maternal bonding and breastfeeding success.

There are situations where active third stage management is necessary, such as when the mother has experienced heavy bleeding during labor, has had twins, or has a history of retained placenta, which significantly increase the risk of postpartum hemorrhage. In these cases, 'modified active third stage management' can be used, which combines active and natural management and allows for delayed cord clamping. It is important to discuss delayed cord clamping with your healthcare provider, especially if active third stage management is needed. Some 'baby-led' hospitals have even started leaving the cord intact if the baby requires immediate medical attention, such as resuscitation, by placing the baby on the bed next to the mother or on her thigh. This is especially important for premature babies, who need a larger bolus of blood from the placenta than full-term babies.

Physiological third stage management allows the placenta to be delivered naturally without medical intervention. Just as during labor, the mother requires a quiet, dark, and relaxed environment for her natural hormones to work to deliver the placenta, which typically occurs 30 minutes to an hour after the birth of the baby. Placing the baby on the mother's chest to initiate breastfeeding can promote the release of oxytocin, which helps contract the uterus and expel the placenta. The baby remains attached to the umbilical cord, allowing oxygen-rich blood to perfuse the baby. Keeping the umbilical cord attached during delivery of the placenta is also beneficial to the mother, as it prevents separation and can help prevent complications during delivery of the placenta, as the natural hormones can work to fully expel it. If cut before the delivery of the placenta, at least two to three minutes should be allowed before cutting the cord. There is a physical change in the cord from when it is engorged with blood to when it becomes white, deflated, and ceases to pulsate. Waiting until the cord has stopped pulsating is a good length of time to allow all the benefits of delayed cord clamping.

Chapter 8: Birthing Options

It's important to choose a health professional and a hospital or birth center that both align with your own personal philosophy of birth. Having the right environment and support from like-minded people will make it substantially easier to achieve a natural, unmedicated birth. No matter where you choose to give birth or with whom, it's important to carefully review their protocols and ideas about natural birth.

Questions to ask your healthcare provider:
- What is the c-section rate at this hospital?

- What do you consider to be a natural birth?
- Do you allow freedom of movement during labor and birth?
- Can I have a water birth or use the shower?
- Are there any time restrictions for labor?
- How do you feel about drug-free labor and birth?
- Do you prefer active or physiological third stage labor?
- Do you believe in delayed cord clamping?

It's important to discuss these and other questions with healthcare providers. If your values for a natural birth do not align, it's okay to shop around and see other providers. You have the right to change providers at any time during your pregnancy. Not all obstetricians and midwives have the same approach; in general, midwives are taught a more natural approach to labor and delivery, while obstetricians are trained to handle medical emergencies and may take a more medicalized approach to all births, regardless of risk. However, there will be midwives who favor medical interventions and obstetricians who favor hands-off natural birth. No matter how hard you plan for a natural, non-medicated birth, if you don't have a provider who is there to facilitate your needs, it will be difficult. Take your time and shop around to find the provider that suits your needs.

There are several options for care and where to give birth in Australia:

- **Public Hospitals** - A large population of woman in Australia will give birth in a public hospital. In Australia, rates of caesareans, and medical interventions in labor in a public hospital are lower than that of a private hospital. It is interesting to know within the public hospital you have a few options for your care.
  - o **Midwifery group practice** - Within some Public hospitals there are Midwifery group Practices (MGP) that operate inside the main

hospital but are separate to the main labor ward. They create a calm homelike environment within the hospital so you can achieve a natural birth with minimal interventions. These practices are run and provide care from midwives who offer a more holistic approach to your birth offering the same midwife throughout your pregnancy, birth and after care. These centres within the hospital offer the safety net of doctors, specialised equipment and medical intervention if needed. Having medical interventions such as emergency caesareans, epidurals, or forceps being a "last case scenario" rather than something that is the standard protocol is a great quality of MGPs. Birth centres often pushes the beds off into the corner so you have freedom to move around and labor in different positions.

The benefit of giving birth with MGP is they have a much lower rate of interventions and a better rate of satisfaction in mothers than the standard labor ward in the public hospital. In uncomplicated births they encourage woman to discharge home four hours after the birth of the baby. This provides a benefit of minimising time spent in hospital especially with current pandemic concerns. These practices are often equipped with the option to have a water birth which is another major draw towards this care method. MGPs often have long waiting list. You must apply to the MGP early in your pregnancy by calling into your local practice to secure a place. This shows many women prefer this way of giving birth but there is limited government funding. The more woman applying and using the

MGP will make more funding for this natural approach to giving birth.

- o **Labor ward with Midwives/Obstetricians** - A woman with a non-complicated labor in a public hospital will generally see midwives during her pregnancy. Unlike the MGP there will be less continuity of care and you will see several different midwives during your antenatal visits. Obstetricians will only be seen when the women is experiencing complications. The view of what a natural birth is and the need for medical interventions will vary from caregiver to caregiver meaning that it is possible to have a completely intervention free birth here but you must have a solid birth plan (Please see example birth plan below) and a good support person with you.

- **Private Hospital** - Private hospital labor and maternity wards are obstetrician led meaning there are no midwifery led care models. Doctors and medical interventions are valuable and can save lives however if you choose to give birth using an obstetrician make sure you have the same definition of what constitutes a natural birth. It may mean to them a vaginal birth where the mother is laboring on bed with an epidural and is delivered by the doctor. It is interesting to note that the rate of caesareans with private obstetricians increases substantially in the days before a long weekend or a big conference. There were also many cases of doctors telling pregnant woman who have had an uncomplicated pregnancy to book to be induced during the height of pandemic lockdowns to avoid uncertainty during the pandemic restrictions. This is not to say you cannot have a non-medicalized birth with an obstetrician, however you must remember that they see all of the births that turned into emergencies and rarely see natural birth as midwives are able to handle the whole labor without them.

Most people do not know that even if you have private insurance you do not have to give birth in a private hospital. It is your right to birth where you choose to meaning you can still opt to birth in a MGP, home or even with private midwives if you choose.

- **Home Birth** - Home births are also on the rise as more and more woman want to move away from the medicalized view of birth. Being in the comfort of your own home can help you to achieve a calm natural birth free of medical intervention. When making the choice to home birth there are several considerations you must make such as factoring in your distance from a hospital if something were to go wrong and ability to have a midwife or obstetrician on call for your birth. Depending on where you live will dictate the availability of homebirth services. It is very important to have a qualified provider at your birth to be there in case any issues should arise.

No matter where you choose to give birth, if you have a support person who is there to help facilitate a natural birth you will be more likely to have the birth you planned for. Having a provider who is there to suggest different positions, relaxation techniques or just being reassuring to get you through it will make all the difference. However, if you have someone who is thinking time is money and suggesting interventions to speed things along you could end up with a cascade of medical interventions and a birth you didn't want. It is very hard to make decisions in the throes of labor which is why your doctor, midwife and support people need to be on the same page as you so they can help you achieve the birth you want. This is when a good birth plan comes into play. Take your time and go through it with your healthcare provider. Sometimes you can have a different doctor or midwife at your birth than who cared for you during your pregnancy. This is why it is important to bring a copy of your plan with you to your place of birth so everyone involved is aware. This is when your partner can be a good spokesperson on your behalf.

For those who do not have a suitable birth partner or wants the support of a seasoned pro, hiring a Doula can be highly beneficial. A Doula is not a midwife or a doctor but someone who has much experience helping laboring woman. She can be there for emotional support, guiding you through your labor and can act as a spokesperson to ensure your medical support people are on the same page as you. Doulas are highly advantageous for woman who might not have a mother, sister or grandmother for maternal support. In today's society where families can be separated by large distances or even when your family lacks the same natural birthing philosophy as you, Doulas can be a fantastic asset.

Example Birth Plan

Your birth plan should be short and concise, no longer than one A4 page. You want doctors and midwives to read this plan, especially those who may not have cared for you during your pregnancy. Having a birth plan does not mean you are inflexible, but it allows others to know how you want your birth to progress. Hopefully, you are in a place that shares your values for natural birth, in which case a birth plan may not be necessary. If this is not the case, a birth plan that summarizes your expectations can be helpful. Below is an example that you can use as a guide to create your own birth plan by adding or removing details.

My Birth Plan
Goal: Calm, natural and unmedicated water birth

***All requests are made within reason. Baby's safety comes first and we are happy for any medical interventions to be made if they are medically required in an emergency situation or situation where the baby or mothers health is compromised.*

During Labor

- My partner will be at the birth
- Water birth with baby birthed in tub
- No IV unless medically indicated / required
- Pain relief: will use meditative and relaxation techniques
- Please re-frain from asking about pain scale
- No epidural or opioid use. Please do not suggest medicated pain control methods
- Please maintain a quiet atmosphere with dim lights and minimal people present
- Freedom of movement and use of rebozo and birthing ball
- Use of mother-directed breathing. Please no "pushing" coaching
- No vaginal exams unless absolutely necessary
- If labor stalls, I would like to try alternative measures before use of Pitocin such as nipple stimulation and movement first

After Birth

- Delayed cord clamping until cord stops pulsating
- After the birth, I would like immediate skin to skin contact and initiation of breast feeding
- Please delay procedures on baby to facilitate bonding and breastfeeding

- Baby-led attachment for breastfeeding. Please give us time and do not assist unless asked
- For delivery of the placenta: no Pitocin unless signs of haemorrhaging or taking longer than one hour to deliver (I wish to use natural oxytocin release from breastfeeding first)
- Early discharge (four hours after birth) from hospital after an uncomplicated natural birth

Chapter 9: When to go to the Hospital

It can be confusing to read about the stages of labor and worry about when to go to the hospital. Signs of labor, such as losing the mucous plug, water breaking, and having loose stools, can happen at any time during labor or not at all for some women. When you go into labor, especially if it's your first baby, it can take a long time. It's important not to rush to the hospital at the first sign of contractions. This is a good time to make sure your bag is packed, have some nourishing food and drink, and take a walk. If you go into labor at night, it's a good idea to try to sleep. This might sound odd, but early labor contractions can often be light and far apart, so if you can sleep through some of it, do it. Make sure your partner sleeps too, as you will need them to be fresh and energetic to assist you during the active phase of labor.

Stay at home as long as you can, unless you live far away from the hospital or clinic where you're giving birth. In that case, consult with your midwife or doctor on the best plan for you. Laboring at home will allow you to be calm and relaxed, which will help labor progress smoothly. The hospital environment can be noisy and scary for some women, which can slow the rate of labor. Hopefully, you are in a good midwifery-run environment where they already have the lights dim, soft music, and limited distractions. If this is not the case, when you get to the hospital, it doesn't hurt to ask them to dim the lights, close the door, and put on headphones with your choice of soothing music so your labor can pick up again.

If you live near the place where you will give birth, you can stay at home until active labor begins. This is when contractions come every three minutes for at least ten minutes. Try not to focus too much on constantly checking your contractions. You will feel when labor progresses into the active stage. If you feel like the labor is coming on too fast and want to slow it down, try getting into a head-down, bottom-up position. This is also a good position to take in the car on the way to where you are giving birth, in case you think the baby will be born on the way. It is very rare for a woman not to make it to her birthing place, so don't worry too much about it. However, it is interesting to note that complications for women who have their babies on the side of the road are very low, because the birth happens so quickly. It's also a good idea to put the car seat in the trunk of the car, so you can ride in the back seat and find a more comfortable position on the way to the hospital.

Water breaking can occur at any time during labor, and some women's waters don't break until the baby is born, while others have babies born with the sack still intact. So, don't rush to the hospital when your waters break. Consult with your healthcare professional, as most hospitals have policies of inducing labor 24 hours after the water breaks to reduce the risk of infection. This also means that after your water breaks, you should avoid anything going into the vagina, and no baths unless they have been properly cleaned beforehand to prevent infection.

Many women make the mistake of going to the hospital too early in their labor. If you go into labor during the day, it is best to continue doing what you were doing. If you were gardening, keep gardening. If you were shopping, keep shopping. Whatever you were doing or planning to do, keep doing it. This will help keep you distracted and moving, which can help labor progress smoothly and easily.

It can be tempting to go and announce to everyone that you are in labor and about to have a baby. However, it is best not to tell anyone you are in labor until you are ready to go to the hospital. Once the news is out, you will have a constant stream of people checking on your progress, which can cause pressure and take away your or your partner's focus while you are in labor. Only inform those who are instrumental in the process, such as your partner or others helping during labor.

The main takeaway from this section is to stay at home as long as possible. Time is of the essence in the hospital, so if you go in too early, you may be told to go home or put on the clock, which increases the likelihood of medical interventions. Staying home will also help you feel more relaxed and less inhibited in your own environment, which is essential for having an easy, natural birth. Choosing a hospital or birth center where you feel safe and relaxed can make all the difference in your labor progress.

Chapter 10: Labor

If you have read the first few chapters of this book, you should have already spent the last nine months preparing your mind and body for labor. By going into labor with a plan and using positive thinking and visualization, you will be able to cope with and manage the mental and physical endurance needed to give birth. The preparation you do during pregnancy is the key to a successful natural birth. This section will give you helpful tips on what to do during labor and birth.

It is interesting to know that sensation during an uncomplicated labor only lasts as long as the contraction last and disappears in between. It can be tiring, but this is why you have prepared and conditioned your body by doing exercises and getting it ready for this moment. The time in between contractions is a time to rest and relax your mind and body so you are prepared for the next contraction. As soon as the baby is out and in your arms, your body and mind have a way of making you forget the journey you just experienced, which is why many women have gone on to have more children. Labor will involve some level of pain and discomfort, depending on the individual, but your perception of this pain will be shaped by your outlook.

In labor, practicing visualization will help you achieve a natural birth. You must first make sure you have a positive mindset. Each contraction should be visualized as bringing you one step closer to having your baby in your arms. Every contraction brings you closer to your baby. If you go into labor thinking that you are going to be in agonizing pain, need an epidural, and have a cesarean, that is most likely what you will get. However, if you go into it with a positive and calm attitude, you are more likely to have the natural birth you have planned for.

The more detail you visualize during labor, the greater effect you will achieve. By focusing your mind on the natural birth you want, you will send oxygen and energy to the area you visualize. It will also focus your mind on the positive end goal of labor instead of fixating on your discomfort.

Below are some images to visualise as you birth your baby:

- Visualise your uterus contracting strongly and effectively to help move your baby easily through the birth canal
- Visualise your body being perfectly designed to give birth
- Visualise your cervix opening so the babies head can pass through easily
- Imagine all of your muscles relaxing in your pelvis
- Imagine your baby in the perfect, anterior position easily passing down your birth canal into your arms
- Visualise your baby gently emerging from your womb into your arms
- Imagine their face, their small nose, tiny hands and feet
- Feel the sensation of your baby against your chest
- Visualise your tiny baby easily finding your breast and begin to nurse

- Visualise yourself, your partner and your baby curled up in bed resting peacefully.

Having a positive end in sight can greatly shape your perception of labor. Make yourself feel excited to hold your baby. You are having contractions and going through labor so that you can meet your baby, whom you have been dreaming of for the last nine months.

Breathing and Relaxing

Breathing and actively relaxing your body are integral to having a smooth and easy birth. The most important thing is to actively relax your muscles. If you clench your muscles during a contraction, your baby will have a harder time coming out. It is a reflex to clench your muscles when you feel pain, but you must try to override this response. Relaxing your muscles during each contraction will decrease your perception of pain during labor and make it shorter and easier. Even women in comas are able to give birth because their uterine contractions can bring the baby out without the mother "pushing." This demonstrates that if you can let go of your fear of labor and allow your body to relax, it can do what it is designed to do.

To relax your muscles during a contraction, you must breathe through it. Holding your breath and clenching your muscles will increase your perception of pain. Remember that pain is in the mind. Your body is designed to give birth to your baby. Labor is not meant to cause pain. It is extremely important to prepare your mind during pregnancy. The more you practice relaxing your mind and body during pregnancy, the easier it will be to relax during labor. There are many different breathing techniques, and any one that works for you is valid and worth trying. The easiest method is to just slow your breathing as much as possible. This will activate your body's parasympathetic nervous system, which, in simple terms, helps relax your body and override the fight or flight response caused by fear and stress. This feeling of calm and relaxation from slow breathing can be enhanced by adding comfort measures such as soaking in the bath, massage, aromatherapy, and laughter.

The Importance of Feeling Unobserved

Women need to feel calm and unobserved during labor. If a cat feels any sense of danger, its body will stop the labor so it can run to a safer location to resume giving birth to its litter. Humans are similar, and will experience a lull in labor when they feel fear. This is why it is common for women to have a stall in labor upon arriving at the hospital. This is why it is vital for the birthing woman to feel unobserved, calm, and relaxed in her birthing environment. Dimming the lights, asking people who do not need to be there to leave, playing soothing music, and meditating are all ways to reinstate a feeling of calm so that labor can progress. If you are familiar with your place of birth, your doctor or midwife, and there is an atmosphere that fosters an unobserved labor, you will be able to quickly get back into the mindset to birth your baby. If this is not the case, you must stand up for yourself and request changes. Your partner or support person should have an integral role in making this happen.

Here are some ideas to create a calm birthing environment:

- **Dim lighting**: Women and animals all feel more calm and relaxed in a dimly lit room. This will be a calmer way for your baby to enter the world as well. Bright fluorescent light will be jarring and confronting for a newborn. Oxytocin is more effective at night-time meaning that creating a dimly lit room will enhance oxytocin release. If you are birthing in the day you can pull curtains and close doors to minimise light.

- **Privacy and feeling unobserved**: Have a "do not disturb" sign on the door. Ensure curtains are drawn and only the people who need to be there are there. It is in your right to ask excessive staff or students to leave. If you feel like you could not hug or kiss your partner in this room, there is not enough privacy and you need to make it into an environment where you feel unobserved and relaxed.

- **Organize the room:** Move beds and equipment so it suits your needs. The bed can be pushed in the corner so you can have more floor space. Yoga mats can be placed on the floor to protect your knees, birthing/exercise balls, chairs, stools can be put out. Aromatherapy oils, music players, affirmations, pictures; anything that you need to get your through labor should be organised in the room so you feel comfortable.

- **Cover clocks:** You do not need to be on the clock in labor. This is distracting and takes your focus away from your birth.

Activities to do During Labor

Below are some activities that you can do at any stage of labor, either before you go to the place where you will give birth or during active labor, to make the process easier:

- **Distraction:** Watch funny movies to relax and take mind off of labor during the early stages of labor. Laughter releases oxytocin which will enhance labor. Pick the funniest, silliest movies you can to help facilitate the release of oxytocin.

- **Dancing:** dance to your favourite music or slow dance with your partner to help sway baby into an optimal position for birth

- **Sitting on the exercise/birth ball:** moving your hips in small circles will help open your hips and help labor progress. Draping your upper body over the ball while on hands and knees can also be a restful position for labor

- **Rebozo:** The rebozo is a highly valuable tool for both in pregnancy and in labor. Using your rebozo in-between contractions will open your pelvis and relax your ligaments for birth. Use this as much as you can.

- **Forward leaning inversions:** Just like during pregnancy, forward leaning inversions can be beneficial for helping get the baby in an optimal position for birth. It can be beneficial in early labor to perform a forward leaning inversion during the length of a contraction. This can be repeated 2 or 3 times. This will take the pressure of the babies head off of your cervix and allow the baby to move into a better position. The next contraction while in an upright position should make a more effective contraction to help birth your baby.

- **Meditation:** Using guided meditation scripts that you used during pregnancy should help put you into a calm and relaxed state in your labor. Focus on visualising your baby easily being born into your arms. Relax and allow all of your muscles to become like jelly. The more relaxed your mind becomes between contractions the easier the contraction will become. The more relaxed your body becomes the easier the baby can pass through the birth canal into your arms. Preparation is key, the more you practiced in pregnancy, the greater effect you will see in labor. Having guided relaxation that you enjoyed during your pregnancy on headphones or being played in the room during labor can help you focus on relaxing and blocking out all other distractions

- **Water:** having a water birth or even just being in the shower can be an effective pain control method

- **Walking:** walking is one of the best things you can do in labor to decrease laboring time, and help baby get into an optimal position for an easy birth. Walk around the block with your partner or support person or even walk the halls of the hospital if you have to. Just keep moving

- **Visualisation:** during labor visualise your cervix opening like flower, the baby easily sliding down birth canal and into your arms. The more detail you visualise the better. This goes hand in hand with the visualisation practice you preformed in pregnancy. If you think this sounds crazy attempt this kind of relaxation and visualization for your next bowl movement. Visualise your BM easily coming down your colon and into the toilet. You should not have to exert any force or push to have a BM. Bizarre but effective.

- **Freedom of movement:** change positions that make you feel good. If you feel like dancing and swaying your hips do it. Any position that makes you feel good. Listen to your natural instincts. Do not be concerned how you might look, whatever movement or dance that gets your baby out is what you need to be doing in a completely uninhibited state.

- **Breathing:** Use the ***golden thread breath*** to help calm your body and birth your baby. Breathe in a long slow breath and then breath out an even longer slow breath like you are blowing a fine, long thread of gold through your pursed lips. This breath can be used any time during labor and is especially good during contractions to relax you. There are many breathing techniques and all are valid as long as it feels right to you. There is no need to be worried about different breaths for different stages. The breath that is calming for you will be the most effective.

- **Relax your face:** If your face is relaxed your pelvic floor will be relaxed. It is very easy to hold tension in your face during contractions. Have your partner remind you to relax your face by blowing raspberries if your face is getting tense. This will not only relax you're your facial and kegal muscles but it will make you laugh. Being able to laugh in labor is a wonderful experience and will flood your body with endorphins and relax your muscles allowing you to birth your baby easily.

- **Deep kissing:** Deep kissing will relax you as well as open up the birth canal. A loose jaw and mouth directly relaxes your pelvic floor. Not only will deep kissing relax your pelvic floor it will it will create a welcomed distraction and causes a release of oxytocin which will help stimulate labor.

- **Sex:** Sex or even 'outer-course' where you engage in physical acts of affection such as kissing and hugging will increase your natural production of oxytocin which will speed up labor and make stronger and more effective contractions. Semen is also a powerful prostaglandin, which a synthetic version is actually used to induce labor, which can act to increase contractions and dilate the cervix. This might sound like the last thing you might be thinking of in labor but it can be a welcomed distraction as well as having the added benefit of speeding things along.

Water birth

Water birth, where the baby is born into a warm pool of water, is becoming more popular for mothers who want to have a natural birth. The warm water supports and provides natural pain relief for the mother's belly. During a water birth, the woman enters the birthing pool during the active phase of labor and gives birth to the baby in the water. The baby is still connected to the umbilical cord and receives oxygen, and their first breath is not initiated until they are taken out of the water and a reflex is triggered. This can be a smooth and calm way for a baby to be born, as there is less of a transition from the warmth of the womb to the warmth of the water. Many babies born this way do not cry upon being born and remain in a calm, relaxed state as they are brought to their mother's chest.

There are many benefits of having a water birth including:

- Less pain experienced by the mother
- Higher satisfaction rates of the birth
- Higher rate of vaginal births
- Less use of medication
- Lower rates of episiotomy
- Lower rates of sever vaginal tears
- Lower use of artificial hormones
- Can possibly decrease the duration of labor

Not only does the water provide pain relief, it also prevents unnecessary vaginal examinations and checks. Mirrors and flashlights can also be used by midwives to see the baby's head emerging. By being in the water, the mother creates a barrier around herself, allowing her to birth the baby in peace. This, combined with dim lighting, a quiet environment, and a minimal number of people, can help the mother feel unobserved and more able to give birth naturally.

If water birth facilities are not available, hydrotherapy can also be effective. Most birth centers and hospitals have showers that can be used, and running warm water over the back and belly can provide pain relief. Due to the popularity of water birth, facilities are becoming more widely available.

Fathers in Labor

It is important to highlight the importance of fathers during labor. Their presence and support can provide great comfort to the mother during labor. Giving your partner a defined role or job to do during labor can also give them a meaningful and active role, instead of feeling on the sidelines and unable to help.

There are many ways a father can help during labor and birth including:

- Being a strong and level-headed support person who has the ability to maintain calm throughout labor and birth
- Being a spokesperson for the mother to maintain her birth plan and ensure her wishes are followed
- Making sure the room is calm and dimly-lit and that the amount of people coming in and out are restricted
- Reminding the mother to breathe through contractions
- Reminding the mother to keep her face relaxed and encouraging raspberry blowing
- Petting or massaging the mothers back
- Kissing or hugging during or in-between contractions to relax the mother
- Using the rebozo on the mother in between contractions
- Keeping the mother hydrated

The birth of their child and the sight of their partner in labor can be an emotionally exhilarating and exhausting experience for fathers. It is important that fathers take care of themselves during labor and birth so that they are able to support the mother. Having a hospital bag packed with essentials like energy bars, caffeine, hydration, and pain medication can be helpful in keeping them in good shape. Being a support person can be emotionally and physically draining, and although the mother is doing the hard work of giving birth, the father is also going through a transformative period in their life. By showing mutual respect and care, the mother and father can support each other and help the baby be born into a calm and happy family. A hospital bag checklist can be found at the end of this book.

Chapter 11: Immediately Following Birth

The feeling right after having a natural birth is euphoric, as the body's hormones are working perfectly without interference from artificial drugs or hormones. These natural hormones help facilitate bonding between you and your baby, breastfeeding, and the birthing of the placenta. The moment that your baby gazes into your eyes and grasps your partner's finger is one of the greatest moments of your life.

Immediate skin-to-skin contact with your baby will initiate bonding, breastfeeding, the birthing of the placenta, and the release of oxytocin. You may have caught your own baby, or someone else may have caught the baby for you and passed them to you so that you can put the naked baby on your naked chest. This releases endorphins and oxytocin in both you and your baby, facilitating bonding. This is also true for the father. It is important for him to bond and connect with the baby. Whenever the mother is unavailable after the birth, such as when she is showering or getting dressed, the father should take off his shirt and have skin-to-skin contact with the baby, covered with a warm blanket. This is a good routine to maintain throughout the newborn phase. Not only will the mother get much-needed alone time to bathe or rest, but the father will also have priceless bonding time that might not have been possible otherwise. It is important to note that smell helps facilitate bonding, so it is best to avoid strong perfumes, deodorants, or soaps. This does not mean you have to smell bad, as there are effective deodorants, such as salt blocks, that prevent body odor without an artificial smell.

Delivering the Placenta and After-Pains

After your baby is born, you will give birth to your placenta around 30 minutes to an hour after a natural birth. This process is much easier than giving birth to a baby. The best way to facilitate the quick birth of the placenta is to nurse your baby. Naked skin-to-skin contact with the baby and nursing will help the release of oxytocin, facilitate the contraction of the uterus to expel the placenta, and allow you to bond with your baby. The contractions may feel intense, especially after giving birth to a baby, but they will also help contract your uterus back to its previous size. Your midwife will massage your abdomen by pressing down on your womb, which may be unpleasant but helps expel much of the blood and further contract the uterus. They will then do a quick vaginal inspection to check for tears or any other issues. You can hold your baby and nurse during this process. Once the placenta is examined to ensure it is intact and has detached completely, your labor is officially over, and your only job is to rest and care for your newborn. If you are lucky enough to give birth in a birth center, you will have a minimum of four hours before you are sent home. Some people are shocked by the short amount of time a new mother spends in the center after a natural birth, but if you had a drug-free, natural birth with no complications, the safest place for you and your family to rest and bond will be at your home. You will be feeling well and able to walk around.

It takes about six weeks for your uterus to shrink back down to its original size, which is why you may still look a few months pregnant after giving birth until your uterus returns to your pelvis. To do this, your uterus will contract, reducing its size and preventing excessive blood loss. These contractions are nothing like labor contractions, but they can be uncomfortable, especially if this is not your first child. Breastfeeding stimulates these contractions for the first few weeks. When you feel discomfort from these contractions, it can be helpful to visualize what is happening physiologically and be happy that you are making progress in your recovery. You can take comfort measures, such as using a hot compress, self-massaging, and using breathing and meditation techniques you used during labor to ease discomfort.

Chapter 12: Having a Positive Caesarean

Although it is beneficial to avoid a caesarean, it is sometimes unavoidable. Women who end up having an emergency caesarean section or even an elective one due to conditions out of their control can still have a positive experience. It is important to know what to expect if you end up having a caesarean. There will be many people working in the operating theater, and it can feel overwhelming if you are unprepared. When you arrive at the theater complex, you will go through multiple checkpoints where you are asked the same questions about your name, date of birth, etc. This is a safety check that ensures the correct person gets the correct procedure. An anesthesiologist will administer a spinal or epidural anesthetic. This is performed by you sitting or lying down. The doctor will clean your back with very cold alcohol and then perform the spinal or epidural. This will make you numb from the waist down. You will be able to feel pressure and prodding but will not feel sharp pain. The doctors and nurses will check this several times before performing the caesarean. You will have an IV in your arm that is connected to fluids and medications. You will be awake and alert. The nurses will place a sheet in front of you so you cannot see the operation. Some doctors may be happy to lower the sheet so you can watch the birth of your baby once they reach that step if you wish. Your partner will be with you the entire time, dressed in scrubs and sitting by your side.

Once the baby is born, a midwife and paediatrician will be present to take care of the baby. They will show you your baby, assess and weigh them under a heat lamp, and wrap them in a blanket, as it is very cold in the theater. When they are finished, they will give the baby back to you or your partner to hold while the obstetrician sutures you up. After the operation, you will be moved to a different bed and taken to the recovery unit with your baby and partner. A midwife or nurse will be with you to help you recover. You will be able to hold your baby here and start breastfeeding. If everything goes well, you will be in the recovery unit for about an hour before being transferred to the ward where you will stay for the next few days.

This process can seem very fast and overwhelming, but you still have the ability to ask questions and know what is happening at every stage. Most doctors and nurses will be very good at informing you every step of the way. If this is not the case, feel free to speak up and ask for clarification. You have the right to care for your baby as you wish. Some midwives may be overbearing and try to attach your baby to the breast or quickly take your baby to be swaddled and put in the crib. You have the right to tell them that you need space and time to bond with your baby. After a cesarean, you may not have the natural hormone high that occurs during a natural birth. This is a minor disadvantage, but it does not mean you will not be successful at breastfeeding. Many women who have had cesareans have gone on to successfully breastfeed their babies. By spending as much time as possible cradling your naked baby against your naked chest, you can help increase your natural production of oxytocin after a cesarean. Cesarean-born babies may be drowsy after birth due to the effects of the anaesthetic drugs. This is not harmful to the baby, but it may mean they need extra time to initiate breastfeeding. The best solution is to keep them close. Open your hospital gown and place your naked baby (a diaper is fine) on your chest, and cover both of you with a warm blanket. The blanket should provide you with some level of modesty, but remember that you are in the hospital and breasts are nothing a doctor or nurse has not seen before.

It is important to stay with your baby unless they require special care. If they need to be separated from you, it is important that the staff know that no supplementary bottles or pacifiers should be given, as this can interfere with breastfeeding. It may also be tempting to let the midwives on the ward take your baby so you can sleep during your stay. However, even if you are expressing milk for a night bottle for them, this can disrupt breastfeeding and lead to milk supply issues. Rooming in with your baby is now common in many hospitals and allows you to prepare for what caring for your baby at home will be like.

If your baby becomes separated from you and needs to go into the neonatal intensive care unit (NICU), it is important to know that you are still an integral member of their care and recovery. Kangaroo care is a proven method to help stabilize premature babies and other babies in the NICU. Kangaroo care involves naked skin-to-skin contact with the baby while they are in the NICU. This can be done from birth and can be performed even while the baby is connected to monitors and tubes.

Kangaroo care has been shown to have numerous benefits such as:

- Increase survival rates

- Improved thermo-regulation
- Improves cardiorespiratory health
- Improves weight gain
- Reduces procedural pain
- Improves neuro-development

Despite recommendations for its use and known benefits, kangaroo care has been underutilized in some NICUs. If your baby ends up in the NICU, it is important that you begin kangaroo care as soon as possible to improve your baby's outcomes. Both mothers and fathers, as well as volunteers, can perform kangaroo care that will improve your baby's health.

Chapter 13: When Things Do Not Go To Plan

In life, things don't always go according to plan. There are many things that are out of your control during childbirth. You may have every intention of having a natural birth and end up with every medical intervention available. In the end, the only thing you can control is your attitude and ability to adapt to whatever life throws at you. In the end, if you have a healthy baby in your arms, you have accomplished something great. There is no shame in any deviation from your original plan. You have just started a lifelong journey with your baby and your family, so take comfort in the fact that you have years of bonding and growing together as a family ahead of you.

It is very important to discuss contingency plans with your healthcare provider for when things don't go according to the original plan. By discussing possible issues and finding out what the protocols are, you will have an idea of what to expect. This is not being negative or expecting the worst, but preparing your mind for all contingencies so you will feel empowered and in control no matter what life throws at you. Having your partner with you during childbirth to act as your spokesperson by making sure you are fully informed and understand what is happening is also important. Unfortunately, for many medical professionals, they perform medical interventions daily and may not realize the profound effect they can have on people when they fail to fully inform or include the patient in what is happening. Any time a procedure is about to be performed, you have the right to ask about the risks and alternatives so you can be fully informed.

For some women, the experience of giving birth can leave them with trauma that can manifest as depression, anxiety, or feelings of loneliness. One woman can have a perceived "traumatic birth" but, because she has good emotional support, was informed and supported throughout labor and delivery, and had continuity of support at home and in the community, she had a positive experience of birth and motherhood. However, the same woman without support or not being well informed could end up experiencing birth in a negative way. Prevention through support and being an active participant in the birth is the best way to prevent any mental health issues, but this is not always possible. It is OK to feel sad after birth, especially if you or your baby experienced trauma or if you felt out of control and things didn't go as planned, and you are grieving the loss of the birth you didn't have. However, if you are feeling depressed and you feel you are a danger to yourself or to your baby, you need to seek help immediately. More commonly, a woman feeling traumatized by birth will struggle in silence.

If you don't feel good after the birth of your baby, you need to seek help. Many women who are experiencing negative emotions after birth are treated with a "band-aid" approach and given antidepressants. If you don't feel right about it in any way, seek additional medical advice or support. Counseling, therapy, and support groups made up of other mothers who are struggling are all beneficial ways of finding someone to listen and offer validation. Often, when women experience trauma, they just want to be heard and validated. Only share your birth story and issues with someone you know will be supportive and will listen when you are feeling down. This is why seeking a counselor or going to support groups can be more beneficial than talking to friends or family who might not understand what you are going through. As well as seeking validation and discussing your reasons for being sad, it is important to invest heavily in your own self-care. Prioritizing your nutrition, rest, exercise, and relaxation will benefit you mentally, physically, and allow you to better care for your new baby.

Please read the following section for tips on improving your physical and mental health during the first six weeks.

PART III – POSTPARTUM

This chapter covers how to take care of yourself and allow your body to heal so you can care for your baby. The concept of postpartum care has been lost in Western countries, causing many new mothers to struggle unnecessarily. This chapter will cover postpartum care, asking for help, diet, and sex after giving birth. I want women to enjoy having a newborn. These should be the happiest days of your life that you can look back on as a time of calm and rest. By respecting your body and asking for support, you can prevent yourself from becoming the stereotypical sleep-deprived and overwhelmed mother of a newborn.

Chapter 14: The First Six Weeks

The first six weeks after the baby is born are an important time for the new mother to rest and recover from pregnancy and childbirth. Many cultures all over the world believe in the philosophy of a six-week or longer period of rest, during which the new mother eats nourishing food and is relieved of all responsibilities besides caring for her baby. In contrast, Western countries seem to have adopted the opposite doctrine and there is a culture of taking pride in getting back to work and not being phased by childbirth as a badge of honor. If a new mother fails to rest and fully recover after giving birth, chronic lethargy called postpartum fatigue can plague her for up to a year or longer after childbirth and can even manifest as other unwanted ailments such as depression and illness. There should be no shame in resting and recovering after giving birth. Don't feel any societal pressure to be out and about if you're not feeling up to it. In some cultures, there is a belief that if the new mother commits to a period of rest after birth, she will recover to a state better than she was before pregnancy.

Chapter 15: Asking for Help

One of the most important things a new mother can learn to do is to ask for help. There seems to be a toxic trend among young mothers to show how they can bounce back very quickly after birth. Even if you are feeling great after a natural birth, it is still important to allow yourself to rest and avoid burnout from over-exerting yourself. Giving birth can give some people a natural high. However, your body still has a lot of work to do to get itself back to how it was, and you have to respect this time of rest. Ask for help as much as you can from friends and family. Everyone wants to come and see the baby. Feel free to say no to these visitors if you need to sleep, or better yet, allow them to come and put them to work. People love babies and genuinely want to help you. Asking for small favors, such as doing the dishes, laundry, or running the vacuum, means you won't have to exert yourself on less important chores. Ask for someone to hold the baby so you can have a shower or take a nap. Ask for people to prepare some healthy food for you or to run to the grocery store for you. Ask for as much help as you can so you can focus on what matters most, which is caring for your baby and allowing yourself to heal and become revitalized.

In the first six weeks after birth, you should sleep when the baby sleeps so your body can heal and recover from pregnancy and childbirth. Everyone will tell you this, but many people fail to follow it. Even if you can't sleep, taking time to turn off your phone, get your book, and curl up in bed or your nursing chair with a herbal tea and a snack will be more beneficial to your health than cleaning the house or mindlessly scrolling through your phone. You can easily clean the house while the baby is awake by putting them in a carrier and narrating what you are cleaning. The baby will love being close to you and hearing your voice. While they are sleeping, you should take the opportunity to rest. The dirt will always be there for you to clean later. Just like during pregnancy, make sure you indulge in true rest. Sitting on your phone or watching TV does not allow your brain to get the rest it needs to make a full recovery after birth.

Chapter 16: Your Morning Routine

It is beneficial to establish a good morning routine with your new baby. Some people may find it difficult to balance their own self-care with caring for a newborn. Without a routine, it can be easy to find yourself in the afternoon without having showered or even changed your clothes. If you are lucky enough to have a partner at home in the mornings, take advantage of it. Have your partner take off his shirt for skin to skin and spend some time bonding with the baby on the couch while you go and have a shower, wash your face, moisturize, fix your hair, change into fresh lounge clothes, and sit down to eat breakfast. Of course, this is an ideal scenario and many women may find themselves alone with a newborn who screams when they are put down.

In these cases, it is still possible to balance caring for a newborn and taking care of yourself in the morning. When you wake up with the baby, prioritize drinking a large glass of water and then attend to the baby's needs. Change their diaper, nurse them, burp them, and spend a few moments bonding with them. Fill their emotional needs by cuddling, caressing, and singing to them. If you are lucky, a newborn might be ready to fall asleep again by the time you have completed all of these tasks. If not, you can take them into the bathroom with you and put them in a safe place to lie, such as a bouncer or on some baby blankets on the floor. Continue to talk and sing to them while you shower and get ready. Sometimes, you may find that this is not working and the baby does not want to be out of your arms. That is fine, take a deep breath and pick up your baby to calm them. You can try again later or proceed to breakfast and try again after eating. I suggest having easy-to-eat breakfast options such as overnight oats or smoothies that you can prepare while holding the baby in a wrap or in your arms, to make your morning routine as easy as possible. It can be easy to always put the baby first and forget about yourself, but prioritizing your own self-care will allow you to care for your baby better because you will be calmer, happier, and mentally prepared for caring for your baby.

Investing in one or two comfortable but stylish lounge outfits will help you feel put together and look fresh in the first weeks after having a baby. Instead of wearing tattered old pyjamas or frumpy, oversized clothes, invest in something that makes you feel and look good. Lounge clothes are not pyjamas; they are not clothes you go out in. They are clothes to wear at home that are comfortable and stylish. I recommend choosing clothes made of natural fabrics such as cotton, linen, or bamboo viscose. Luxurious-feeling fabrics will automatically make you feel good. Choose something that is loose and comfortable that you can nap in and that allows you to nurse comfortably. Having a stylish outfit to wear while you stay home with the baby will allow you to receive visitors without feeling slatternly. In addition, it is good for your own mental health to be presentable and get cleaned and dressed in the morning. There is nothing worse than realizing you are still wearing three-day-old pyjamas that smell of old milk. Use one of your baby's muslin blankets as an all-purpose burp cloth that you keep over your shoulder for unavoidable spit-ups. By practicing daily self-care and looking after both your appearance and mind, you will feel and look good.

Making time each day to get out of the house for a walk is an important part of maintaining your self-care. Not only is this beneficial for your mental and physical well-being, it will be beneficial for your newborn to see, smell, and feel the sensations of being outside. By putting your baby in a carrier and going for a relaxing stroll every morning, you can provide them with new experiences and give them the opportunity to see the world through you. Depending on how you feel and where you are in your recovery, this can be as simple as walking around the block or in your backyard, or making your way to the park or beach for a walk. Bringing a picnic blanket and a book is a lovely way to spend time with your newborn. You can place them on the blanket so they can gaze at the scenery. Sitting in the shade under a tree with your baby gazing up at the leaves is a great sensory stimulus for them. Your baby might even drift off to sleep on the blanket, allowing you both to have a much-needed nap and rest. Taking breaks like these will break up the monotony of staying home all day while still respecting your body and allowing you to rest and recover after birth.

Chapter 17: Postpartum Diet

During the first six weeks after birth, it is important to eat easily digested and nourishing food to help you regain your energy and vitality. This is not about losing weight or looking good, but rather about supporting your health and long-term recovery. By prioritizing your health, you may also see changes in your appearance. There is also a physiological reason to eating easily digestible food. During pregnancy, your organs, including your intestines, shift inside your abdomen to make room for your growing baby. After you give birth, it takes time for your uterus to return to its original size and for your intestines to return to their original position. Constipation, wind, and intestinal discomfort are all common issues faced after giving birth. By eating whole foods with an emphasis on hydration, you can help avoid these complications. Many private hospitals boast of giving new mothers steak and a glass of champagne on the last night in the hospital, but this is possibly the worst food a new mother could eat as red meat and alcohol are very hard to digest.

Many cultures have traditional postpartum foods that new mothers eat that are nourishing and easy on their stomachs. Koreans serve new mothers a seaweed soup, Chinese women are given warm congee and sweet red date teas, and Mexican women avoid spicy foods and indulge in warm broths and herbs that help milk production. The common element in these traditional meals is that they are all home-cooked, made of whole foods, and high in fluids. Maintaining hydration after birth is extremely important. By maintaining hydration through drinking warm drinks, soups, and easy-to-digest foods, you will be allowing your intestines to heal. Please see below for recipes for these traditional meals and some other simple whole food meals that will help you recover after birth.

Sample recipes for the first six weeks:

Korean Seaweed Soup 'Miyeok Guk'

This soup is a traditional postpartum meal for new mothers in Korea. It has numerous health benefits as it is low in calorie while being high in iodine, calcium, omega oils and B vitamins. It is said to increase milk supply and speed up postpartum recovery as it detoxifies the body and improves metabolism. This soup is high in fibre as well as having a large fluid content making it easy to digest while maintaining hydration in the new mother. Koreans will traditionally consume this soup several times a day for the first month postpartum. This warm and comforting soup is easy to prepare and is a great staple to add to your postpartum diet.

Ingredients

- 1 oz. Dried brown seaweed/wakame (ensure you have plain dried seaweed. Not the kind you make sushi with or the seasoned seaweed in small packages. It can be found in Asian grocery stores. The seaweed is dried in its original state and only have 'seaweed' listed on the ingredient list. Inside the package you can see the dried seaweed looks like long tangled masses of dried dark green or brown leaves.
- ¼ cup of dried shitake mushroom (can use fresh if you have it)
- 1 cup of stock of choice. Traditionally beef stock is used but can be easily made with
  Vegetable or other stock
- ½ tsp. of minced garlic
- 1Tbs of fish sauce or soy sauce

- 1 tsp. sesame oil
- 4 cups of water plus more for soaking the seaweed

Method

- Place seaweed into in a large bowl and submerge in cold water. Allow to soak until soft. You can soak overnight if you wish. If you do not have a kitchen scale 1 ounce of dried seaweed is roughly a large handful.
- Rinse and drain seaweed
- Cut up the seaweed into bite size pieces
- In a large pot add the sesame oil and heat
- Add garlic to the pot and fry until aromatic, approximately 1-2 minutes
- Add soy sauce and seaweed and fry an additional 2 minutes
- Add the stock, water and dried mushrooms and simmer for 10 minutes
- Turn off heat and allow soup to

Serve with some roasted sesame seeds sprinkled on top. This will yield approximately eight serves. Leftovers can be saved in the fridge to be consumed over the next few days.

Chinese red date tea

This traditional postpartum drink is used by Chinese woman to speed up their postpartum recovery. This drink is sweet, warm and can be sipped from a thermos throughout the day to maintain hydration and provide nourishment. Chinese red dates also known as jujube are high in vitamins A, B1, B2 and C, contain protein, calcium, phosphorous, iron, magnesium and antioxidants. This is a great tea to request any visitors or your partner to make for you while you nurse your baby. Make this daily and drink as you would water.

Ingredients

- 2 cups of Dried Chinese red dates/jujube; can be found in Asian grocery stores. Can buy whole or chopped up
- ¼ cup Dried goji berries; can be found in most grocery stores as well as Asian grocers
- 7 cups of Water

Method

- If using whole red dates remove seeds and chop up
- Add red dates to a large pot with water
- Bring to the boil then reduce heat to a simmer and cover with lid
- Simmer for one hour
- Add dried goji berries and simmer for 30 minutes longer
- Strain and add to a large thermos and sip throughout the day

Congee

Congee is a traditional postpartum meal for new mothers. It is hydrating and easy to digest. It can be made to suit your taste by adding or subtracting additional ingredients. This is an ideal postpartum food in its simplicity. It can be easily cooked in a rice cooker or slow cooker or on the stove.

Ingredients

- 1 cup rice
- 7-8 cups water
- Additional ingredients include
- Dried seaweed
- Dried mushrooms
- Ginger
- Garlic
- Soy sauce

- Chinese red dates and goji berries to make a sweet congee
- Nuts and seeds
- Broths

Method

- Place the rice and water in your cooking method of choice and cook until soft and the rice takes a watery porridge like consistency.

Smoothies

A smoothie might not be a traditional postpartum food however it has a place as a modern woman's postpartum staple. Easy to and quick to make as well as having the benefit of being as nutritionally complete as you would like to make it. By adding in protein powders, green leafy vegetables, cooked beans, nuts and seeds you can make it as a high protein meal or as simple as your taste would like. Below is a basic smoothie recipe that you can easily adjust to your needs.

Ingredients

- 1 large ripe banana
- 1 Tbs of pepita seeds
- 1 Tbs of natural nut butter of choice
- 1.5 cup of milk or plant milk of choice
- 1 tsp of honey or maple syrup

Method

- Place all ingredients in a blender and blend until smooth

Oatmeal

This is another modern woman's postpartum staple. Oats are known to be beneficial in increasing milk supply as well as being high in fibre, iron and antioxidants. They are very easy to digest and can be mixed with many foods to change the flavour depending on your taste. Try adding nuts, seeds, nut butters, apples, bananas and spices such as cinnamon and nutmeg. This nutritious meal does not need to be confined to breakfast and can be eaten at any time during the day or night.

Ingredients

- 1:2 ratio of oats:water depending on how hungry you are you can make anywhere from 1/3 cup oats to 1 cup
- Toppings: bananas, honey, almond butter, chia seeds, pepita seeds

Method

- Add oats and water to a pot on stove and cook on low heat until soft
- Serve in bowl with toppings. Adding a splash of milk or plant milk to the cooked oats can make a creamier consistency

Caffeine

There are many old wives' tales that the kind of food you eat can make your baby fussy. Many women unnecessarily avoid certain foods such as garlic, spicy foods, or allergy-inducing foods like peanuts while breastfeeding. However, there are some considerations to make when it comes to your diet while nursing your baby.

It is not widely known that caffeine has an almost 80-hour half-life in newborns. It is generally safe for mothers to consume caffeine in moderation, but some newborns can be highly sensitive to caffeine and a mother having just one cup of coffee can stay in their system for days. If you're wondering how you can manage a new baby without caffeine, you might be surprised to know that there is evidence to show that regular coffee drinkers are no more alert than non-coffee drinkers. Coffee drinkers are more likely to be staving off caffeine withdrawals than having a genuine energy boost. If you adhere to an initial six weeks of rest where you sleep when the baby sleeps and take care of yourself, you will find you have plenty of energy to look after your baby.

Caffeine can also have a negative effect on iron absorption. Postpartum iron deficiency can occur due to bleeding after birth, making it an important time to increase your iron stores through diet and, if indicated by your doctor or midwife, supplementation. Avoiding caffeine will help improve your dietary absorption of iron. For some, it may be too hard to avoid caffeine entirely. If you do consume caffeine, try to avoid pairing it with iron-rich meals and keep your consumption to a minimum.

Chapter 18: Sex after Birth

Doctors and midwives will often advise against having penetrative sex for six weeks after giving birth, to allow time for the vagina to heal. However, they may not mention that kissing, hugging, touching, and achieving orgasm are all completely safe and should be enjoyed after birth. It took sex to get pregnant, and giving birth is a sexually charged event. Oxytocin, the hormone released during orgasm, is the same hormone released during and after birth to help you bond and fall in love with your baby. It only makes sense that giving birth would heighten your bond with your partner. Engaging in daily affection after birth is important for both you and your partner. Even if you are not feeling sensual after birth or worried about how your body has changed, you should still engage in affection with your partner for a number of reasons. Firstly, having an orgasm will increase blood flow to your vagina and womb, which can help with healing and even help your uterus contract to its previous size. Your partner might be feeling left out as your focus has shifted from him to the baby. Taking time to connect and bond with him will help solidify the bond of your new family dynamic. This doesn't mean working just to please him, it simply means enjoying hugging and being together and doing whatever you feel able to do after birth. Embrace your sexuality after birth and, at a minimum, make sure to hug and kiss your partner every day.

Chapter 19: Contraception

Unfortunately, many practitioners will tell a mother to start taking hormonal birth control immediately after giving birth to prevent further pregnancies without discussing all of the risk factors associated with taking "the pill." Since its conception, the combined pill has been marketed as a way for women to be sexually liberated. Many girls and women are put on the pill without ever being fully informed about the potential side effects.

Some common side effects of the combined oral contraceptive pill include:

- Can alter a woman's sexual preferences in men
- Increases risk of breast cancer
- Increases risk of blood clots
- Can cause mood changes/mood swings
- Weight gain
- Increased use of antidepressants in users
- Alters natural regulation of hormone production
- Decreases testosterone which can lead to decreased calcium stores and poor muscle development

Many breastfeeding women are prescribed the progesterone only 'mini pill' after birth. Unlike the combined oral contraceptive pill, it contains no oestrogen. The mini pill which is given to breastfeeding mothers works by tricking your body into thinking it is pregnant. This means although it carries less risk than the oestrogen-containing pill it carries its own symptoms that mimic many of those in pregnancy.

These include:

- Mood swings
- Swollen and tender breast
- Increased risk of blood clots and stroke
- Not effective if not taken at the same time everyday
- Can have unpredictable breakthrough bleeding

Hormonal contraception can have significant effects on the mental and physical health of women. Many people would not willingly take a drug if they knew it would affect their personalities and sexual identities, but that is what millions of women have done. There has been a loss of knowledge about fertility planning, and it is not surprising that many women struggle to conceive or experience hormonal imbalances when the vast majority are taking a hormonal drug that disrupts their body's production of hormones. Women who use hormonal birth control to regulate their hormones should consider alternative methods, such as diet and exercise. It is important to note that sugar is a major endocrine disruptor. A balanced whole food diet can be beneficial for some women experiencing fluctuating hormones.

Alternative contraception options for lactating women include fertility awareness methods. While these methods are outside the scope of this book, it is important to note that women can take charge of their fertility by tracking their cycles through methods such as basal temperature monitoring, cervical mucus tracking, and period tracking. When used in combination, these methods can be highly effective in preventing pregnancy. You may wish to seek out more information on fertility awareness methods through books at your local library.

It is important to understand that breastfeeding is not a foolproof method of preventing pregnancy. While breastfeeding may temporarily delay your period, it is still possible to ovulate, have intercourse, and become pregnant during this time. Barrier methods such as condoms are effective for preventing pregnancy until your cycle becomes regular again and you can use fertility awareness as a contraception method. Some people may view breastfeeding as a natural way to space out pregnancies, but it is important to be aware that many women who have exclusively breastfed have become pregnant shortly after giving birth. If you choose to use breastfeeding as a means of spacing children, be prepared for the possibility of having children close together, which can also come with many benefits.

PART IV – BREASTFEEDING

This chapter covers an introduction to breastfeeding, including the benefits for mother and baby, attaching the baby to the breast, pumping, common breastfeeding myths, and feeding your baby in public. The goal is to help new mothers feel confident and motivated to breastfeed their babies for as long as they can. It is unfortunate that in Australia, while more than 90% of mothers leave the hospital breastfeeding, by 3 months old, less than 40% of babies are exclusively breastfed. The rate of breastfeeding continues to decline thereafter, falling short of the World Health Organization's recommendations that babies be exclusively breastfed for the first 6 months and continue to breastfeed for at least 2 years and beyond. Through education and increased exposure to breastfeeding, it is hoped that new mothers can successfully nurse their babies.

Chapter 20: Breastfeeding Benefits

Breastfeeding is the best way to nourish and care for your baby as they grow. It is nutritionally superior to any formula and is always easily accessible without the need to get out of bed in the middle of the night or clean up bottles. Additionally, breastfeeding offers numerous benefits for both the baby and the mother.

Benefits for the mother:

- Reduced postpartum bleeding
- Uterus contracts to original size faster
- Helps facilitate postpartum weight loss
- Reduces the risk of postpartum depression
- Facilitates bonding with the baby
- Breastfeeding releases oxytocin which allows the mother to feel relaxed and fall in love with her baby
- Can lower risk of breast cancer
- Can lower risk of ovarian cancer
- Can prevent osteoporosis in old age
- Prevents hypertension and heart disease

Benefits for the baby:

- Builds immunity
- Lower rates of illness
- Lower rate of infant mortality
- Lower rates of sudden infant death syndrome (SIDS)
- Decreases the risk of allergies developing
- Improved neuro-development
- Breastfed babies cry less, meaning a calmer happier baby

For these reasons and more, I would strongly recommend breastfeeding your baby over other methods.

Chapter 21: Initiating Breastfeeding

In today's culture, many women do not grow up seeing babies being breastfed. For many, having a baby is their first time being exposed to breastfeeding. This is why it is important to join a local breastfeeding association or mother's group while you are pregnant. Attending these groups while you are pregnant allows you to experience other women nursing, especially if you have not been exposed to breastfeeding before. This is a beneficial way to normalize nursing and help you mentally prepare for breastfeeding your own baby. Normalizing breastfeeding through contact with nursing mothers is the single best way to prepare yourself for a successful breastfeeding relationship with your child. If animals like cats or cows can naturally feed their babies, you can too. The majority of breastfeeding issues start before the baby is even born, with the mother having fears or misinformation about breastfeeding being difficult. While it may take time to become comfortable and feel confident with breastfeeding, it is a natural process.

The best way to initiate breastfeeding is to allow the baby to self-attach from the first nursing session after birth. Babies have a natural instinct to seek out their mother's breast and, if given the opportunity, will crawl from the mother's belly to the breast to start feeding without any intervention. This process can take up to an hour, but self-attachment can also be achieved by simply cradling the baby in your arms and letting them find the breast without directing them. By allowing the baby as much movement as possible to attach on their own, you will get the best latch. Lying in a reclined position is often an easy way to do this. Self-attachment is beneficial because it provides the best latch and prevents misattachment or nipple damage. Like animals, infants are instinctively able to attach to the breast without intervention.

Sometimes, babies can be quite drowsy after a medicalized birth, depending on the delivery and any drugs that may be in their system. In this case, gentle encouragement can be helpful. Having as much naked skin-to-skin time can help facilitate the first feedings. If the baby is sleepy, simply cradling them in your arms and rubbing your nipple down their nose towards their mouth can help stimulate their natural instinct to open their mouth wide. Once their mouth is open, you can place your breast in their mouth, aiming the nipple over their tongue and down the back of their throat. If you experience any discomfort, detach the baby by inserting your finger in the side of their mouth to break the suction and then removing your breast. Try holding the baby in a different position and allowing them to reattach. A newborn baby has the natural instinct to self-attach for up to six weeks after birth, so it is important to allow them to self-attach as much as possible during this time, even if you have to initially attach them.

After giving birth, your breasts will produce a nutrient-rich fluid called colostrum for the first three to four days. Colostrum helps to build your newborn's immune system and is produced in small amounts. Your newborn will nurse very frequently during this time to establish your milk supply. It is common for newborns to nurse every 30 minutes or more. This frequent nursing helps to stimulate your body to produce more milk. Your breast milk production works on a supply and demand basis, so the more the baby nurses, the more milk will be produced. Breastfeeding on demand, rather than on a schedule, allows your body to produce the right amount of milk for your baby. Scheduled feedings may disrupt milk production and lead to supply issues or mastitis. Initially, your breasts may become engorged due to the body's ability to produce enough milk for multiple babies, as in the case of twins. Pumping after nursing can also stimulate your body to produce more milk, as it may think you are feeding twins.

Chapter 22: Myths about Breastfeeding

There are many myths about breastfeeding that can cause unnecessary struggles for new mothers. These myths can come from various sources, including the internet, misinformed family and friends, and even healthcare providers such as doctors or midwives. It's important to be aware of these myths and to seek out accurate information so that you can make informed decisions about breastfeeding.

Some common myths about breastfeeding include:

- Myth: You must pump after the baby feeds to prevent mastitis and completely drain your breast.
  - Truth: Your body will adapt to make the right amount of milk for your baby, which is why nursing on demand is important in the beginning. Initially, your breasts may overproduce milk and become engorged, but nursing as frequently as your baby needs will help regulate your milk supply. If your breasts are still hard and painful after a feeding, you can try hand expressing a small amount of milk into a towel or shower to relieve the pressure. However, it is not necessary to completely drain your breasts, as this may confuse your body into thinking the baby needs more milk, leading to further engorgement and discomfort.
- Myth: Newborn babies should sleep through the night.
  - Truth: Newborns have small stomachs, so they need to eat little and often, including during the night. One way to make nighttime feedings easier is to have your baby in your room, possibly using a co-sleeper cot. This way, you can nurse lying

down in bed while you are half asleep, rather than getting up to feed your baby.

- Myth: Breastfeeding hurts.
  - Truth: Breastfeeding should not be painful. If it is, try detaching your baby by placing a clean finger in the corner of their mouth to break the seal and allow them to self-attach again.
- Myth: You should avoid certain foods while nursing.
  - Truth: It is true that certain drugs, alcohol, and caffeine should be avoided while nursing, as they can pass into the milk and harm your baby. However, as long as you have a balanced diet that includes a variety of foods, you can introduce your baby to the flavors of your family's diet and prepare them to be a good eater in the future.
- Myth: You cannot produce enough milk for your baby.
  - Truth: Most mothers CAN produce more than enough milk for their babies. Very few women have a medical issue that prevents them from producing milk. The issue is often mental, where some women become fixated on how much milk their babies are getting. It can be difficult for some women to accept that their baby is getting enough milk without knowing the volume they are receiving. Remember that breastfeeding is different from bottle-feeding, where you control the amount your baby drinks. With breastfeeding, the baby is in control. A good rule of thumb is if the baby is content, gaining weight, and having wet and dirty diapers, they are getting enough milk!
- Myth: A baby who nurses often is not getting enough milk.
  - Truth: Babies can nurse for various reasons, including comfort, bonding, affection, or even

boredom. Newborn babies must eat frequently due to their small stomach sizes and to establish their mother's milk supply.

- Myth: You can breastfeed too often.
  - Truth: You cannot nurse too often. Breastfeeding can serve more purposes than just providing food. Breastfed babies can nurse for comfort when they become overstimulated or when they just need to be held. This is a great tool for new mothers to have on hand to calm a fussy newborn. Some people who have never breastfed on demand may not understand that newborns can feed very frequently. Do not let negative comments discourage you from nursing your baby when they need it.
- Myth: I cannot produce any milk when I pump, so I have a low milk supply. Truth: Pumping is not a reliable indicator of milk supply. Many women can successfully breastfeed their babies even if they cannot pump. No pump can compare to a baby's natural nursing reflex.
- Myth: My breasts have become smaller, which means my milk has dried up.
  - Truth: After your milk supply has been established and your breasts are not producing an excess of milk, they will soften and decrease in size from their post-birth, engorged state. Women with small breasts are just as capable of producing sufficient milk as women with larger breasts.
- Myth: You must swap breasts every 15 minutes to avoid mastitis.
  - Truth: There is no need to swap breasts during a feeding unless your baby indicates a desire to do so. It is generally recommended to nurse on one breast per feeding session and then switch to the

other breast for the next feeding. This ensures that both breasts are used equally. You and your baby will naturally know which breast to use. Trust your body's natural instincts and try not to worry excessively.

The most important thing to remember is that simplicity is key. You and your baby are all you need. Try not to overthink it and let your natural instincts guide you. Many breastfeeding issues arise when mothers try to do their best for their babies, but become overwhelmed by all the advice from healthcare providers, family, and the internet, and lose their own inner guidance. The more you allow breastfeeding to be a natural process, the easier it will be to feed your baby.

Chapter 23: Fathers and Breastfeeding

There are many ways that fathers and partners can help establish successful breastfeeding. The most important thing they can do is to be supportive. Attending a breastfeeding class with your partner during pregnancy is a great way to prepare for a successful breastfeeding relationship. By attending together, you can make sure you are both on the same page and normalize breastfeeding for both of you. Some people mistakenly believe that if a woman is breastfeeding, the partner will have less bonding time with the baby and will not be able to contribute to feeding the baby. This is not true. In fact, having a supportive person is key to success in breastfeeding.

There are several ways fathers can help with breastfeeding:

- Keeping the mother hydrated by bringing her drinks while nursing. Investing in a metal straw or a high-quality glass or stainless steel water bottle can make it easier to drink while holding a baby. Fathers can even hold the drink for the mother on occasions when the baby is nursing well and you don't want to disturb them.

- Helping the mother get comfortable nursing by positioning pillows, bringing over a book, covering with a blanket, etc. Nursing can be hard work, so having someone to help the mother feel comfortable can be a great help.

- Splitting baby care shifts to suit your lifestyle. For example, the mother can wake at night to nurse the baby, while the father takes the baby in the morning to allow the mother to sleep longer.

- Having daily "naked skin to skin" time with the baby to facilitate bonding between the father and the baby and to allow the mother some time for self-care.

- Being positive and supportive of breastfeeding, even if the mother is having a bad day. Encouraging the mother and reminding her that she is doing a good job can make a big difference in the long term success of nursing.

Chapter 24: Pumping

There are many reasons why mothers may need to pump, and if using a pump allows you to give breast milk to your baby, that is what is most important. However, it is best to start your breastfeeding relationship with your child as nature intended and nurse exclusively. There is a lot of misinformation about breastfeeding that suggests using a pump to fully drain the breast after the baby feeds or to fix engorgement. While there may be legitimate reasons for pumping, such as returning to work, it is best to avoid pumping until you absolutely need to. Nursing exclusively, if possible during the newborn stage, will set you up for a successful breastfeeding relationship.

Cows in a pasture that are allowed to nurse their calves rarely encounter issues with mastitis. However, dairy cows that are pumped daily often suffer from mastitis, which is why there is an upper limit of pus allowed in supermarket milk. This shows that if there is no strong reason to pump, especially in the first month or so while your milk supply is being regulated, it is best to avoid pumping until you have an established breastfeeding relationship and your body has regulated your supply. If you do need to pump, it can be helpful to seek the assistance of a breastfeeding association or a lactation consultant to make the transition easier.

Chapter 25: Breastfeeding in Public

Many new mothers may feel anxious about breastfeeding in public. This can be very detrimental to their mental health, making them feel isolated and confined to their homes. Fortunately, in countries like Australia, breastfeeding in public is becoming more normalized, with many new mothers nursing openly in public. There may be some older people who are scandalized, as this was not how things were done in the past, but modern mothers have the freedom to breastfeed wherever they please. It is interesting that you can walk into any gas station and see scantily clad women on the covers of magazines or watch TV shows and music videos that border on pornography, but the sight of a breastfeeding mother's nipple is somehow considered scandalous. If you're worried about breastfeeding in public, try nursing in front of a mirror. You may be surprised to see that very little of the woman's breast is exposed, with the baby's head and clothing providing modesty. Don't let fear of breastfeeding in public stop you from being social and going out with your newborn. Going to cafes to eat and catch up with friends while your newborn happily nurses or naps in your arms can be a fun and social aspect of being a new mother.

Chapter 26: Time to Rest

It's important to be prepared for the fact that you will be spending a significant amount of time breastfeeding your baby. It can be easy to start feeling like a human pacifier, but it's important to remember that this time should be utilized. There is no other time in life quite like breastfeeding where you can sit still and be alone with your thoughts. This time can easily be wasted if you take out your phone and mindlessly play games or browse social media. While it's normal to need a brain-deadening escape sometimes, when you look back on all the hours you spent breastfeeding, would you rather remember all the screen time you racked up or be proud of the fact that you caught up on your rest or reading? One item that I highly recommend investing in while pregnant is an e-book. They are easy to hold and read while nursing, whether sitting up or lying down. Not only is reading restful and good for your brain, but you can also read aloud to your baby when you have the energy. It doesn't matter what book you are reading; the baby will love being close to you and hearing your voice. This will also help your baby's language centers in their brain grow. On days when you are busy, especially as your baby gets older, know that feeding your baby in a wrap or carrier is an easy way to feed them and get small chores done at the same time.

CONCLUSION

I wrote this book to provide information that I wish I had when I was pregnant with my first child. I believe that there has been a loss of family and societal support for new mothers and a strong emphasis on independence and the idea of "I can do it all by myself." This has led to a generation of young women who struggle through motherhood without being able to fully enjoy it. Pregnancy and motherhood should be the happiest time in your life.

This book discussed how to have an easy and natural pregnancy and birth by focusing on your mind and body by mentally and physically preparing for birth as you would for a marathon. By focusing on forming strong relationships with your partner, family and making new connections in the community you are setting yourself up for a successful birth and beyond. This book also gave a pragmatic and minimal guide to what you need to purchase for your baby. The cost of raising children can vary depending on how frugal or extravagant you choose to be. The first six weeks after birth are a time to focus on rest and recovery, and to take advantage of any help that is available.

I hope that this book will help women have an easy, calm, and natural pregnancy and birth, and that they go on to become easy, natural mothers. There is no greater gift for a woman than the experience of growing, birthing, and raising a child. A natural birth philosophy during pregnancy and labor can help you become a more calm and natural mother.

It is important to create a calm, happy, and safe environment for your child, and by taking care of yourself and showing yourself love, you can better nurture your children and teach them the values of happiness and self-respect for their mind and their body.

CHECKLISTS FOR THE EXPECTANT MOTHER

This section of the book is designed to provide new mothers with a set of helpful checklists to make their transition into motherhood as smooth as possible. These checklists cover various aspects of motherhood such as prenatal care, postpartum recovery, baby care, and more. By following these checklists, a new mother can feel more organized, less overwhelmed, and better prepared for the journey of motherhood. The goal of the section is to make a new mother's life easier by providing them with tools to help them navigate this new chapter in their lives.

Checklist 1: Postpartum Supplies for Mother

- ☐ Nursing pads (cloth or disposable)
- ☐ Maternity pads
- ☐ Comfortable clothes that allow for breastfeeding
- ☐ Witch hazel for the perineal area, to be applied on maternity pads or directly if there are tears or soreness
- ☐ Ingredients for postpartum meals
- ☐ A quiet and comfortable area in your home, such as a rocking chair or lounge, where you can spend long hours nursing your baby
- ☐ A high-quality water bottle or thermos for sipping water or tea throughout the day (preferably made of glass or stainless steel)
- ☐ An e-book or a large selection of physical books to read

Checklist 2: The Bare Minimum Baby Essentials

- ☐ Baby car seat
- ☐ Baby sleeping space (such as a co-sleeper, bassinet, or family bed)
- ☐ Nappy squares (small, square white towels found in the baby section that can be used for various purposes, including as a burp cloth or diaper)
- ☐ Five short-sleeve onesies
- ☐ Five long-sleeve onesies
- ☐ Five pairs of pants
- ☐ Five pairs of socks
- ☐ Five lightweight cotton swaddles
- ☐ Change table (optional, but can help prevent backaches)
- ☐ Diapers (cloth or chemical free disposable)
- ☐ Reusable wipes or disposable water wipes, tissues, or cotton balls (wipes can contain harmful chemicals or alcohols that are not suitable for newborns. Tissues or cotton balls can be wet and used as wipes)
- ☐ Baby carrier or wrap
- ☐ Stroller/pram; it is not essential to have an expensive bassinet attachment if you use a baby carrier for the first three months
- ☐ Nursing chair

Checklist 3: Your Hospital Bag

Note: It is a good idea to pack for an overnight stay, even if you only plan to be at the hospital or birthing center for a few hours after giving birth. This is because it is always good to be prepared for any unexpected developments, and it is helpful to be able to freshen up and change your clothes before you leave.

- ☐ Rebozo
- ☐ Robe (hospitals can be cold)
- ☐ Slippers
- ☐ Underwear
- ☐ Pajamas
- ☐ Camera
- ☐ Music or guided meditation with corresponding device and headphones
- ☐ Phone and phone charger
- ☐ Energy snacks and water/coconut water for Mom and Dad
- ☐ Going home outfit for Mom:
- ☐ Loose, breathable clothing that allows for breastfeeding
- ☐ Comfortable, large underwear to accommodate maternity pads
- ☐ Toiletries:
  - ○ Facecloth
  - ○ Hair brush
  - ○ Hair tie
  - ○ Toothbrush and toothpaste
  - ○ Deodorant
  - ○ Moisturizer
  - ○ Maternity pads
  - ○ Breast pads
- ☐ For Dad:

- ○ Spare clothes and underwear, including a swim-suit if planning a water birth
- ○ Energy bars or snacks
- ○ Caffeinated drinks
- ○ Phone and charger
- ○ Camera and charger
- ☐ For baby:
  - ○ Two swaddles
  - ○ Two comfortable, easy-to-put-on onesies, suitable for the weather
  - ○ Newborn diapers
  - ○ Water wipes, cotton balls, or reusable wipes

Checklist 4: Things to do Before Your Baby is Born

☐ Set up the car seat (note that it is a good idea not to have it installed in the car on the way to the hospital, in case you need to lie down or kneel in the back of the car)

☐ Plan a date night or "babymoon"

☐ Make arrangements for girls' day out with friends

☐ Make arrangements for pets or older children while you are in labor

☐ Prepare meals for after the birth

☐ Set up the baby's sleeping space

☐ Set up the diaper-changing area

☐ Organize your maternity leave

☐ Clean the house

☐ Write thank you letters for the baby shower

☐ Create a comfortable and calming "nest" for you and your baby, including a nursing chair, table, books, etc.

☐ Make a list of people to notify of the baby's birth

Checklist 5: Packing a Newborn Nappie Bag

- ☐ Bag of your choice (an old backpack can work well)
- ☐ 2 square nappy towels
- ☐ 2 muslin blankets
- ☐ 8 diapers (cloth or disposable)
- ☐ Water wipes or cloth wipes
- ☐ 2 extra outfits, including socks
- ☐ 2 bibs for spit-ups
- ☐ Change mat
- ☐ Nursing pads and maternity pads for the mother
- ☐ Water bottle for the mother

Checklist 6: Daily Exercise and Activities to Promote an Easy Birth

☐ Walk for one hour at a brisk pace

☐ Perform "cat cow" yoga pose on your hands and knees while doing kegel exercises

☐ Do a forward-leaning inversion from the second trimester

☐ Spend 20 minutes on positive birth meditation

☐ Avoid screens for one hour (use this time for rest, reading, sleeping, taking a bath, or pursuing a hobby)

☐ Spend 5 minutes each night using a Rebozo from the third trimester (can be done earlier if desired)

Checklist 7: Weekly Activities to Promote an Easy Birth

- ☐ Have a date night with your partner
- ☐ Scrub floors to promote good fetal positioning (can be done more frequently if desired)
- ☐ Attend a yoga or pregnancy exercise group class
- ☐ Get pregnancy body work from a specialist, such as a chiropractor, physiotherapist, or osteopath

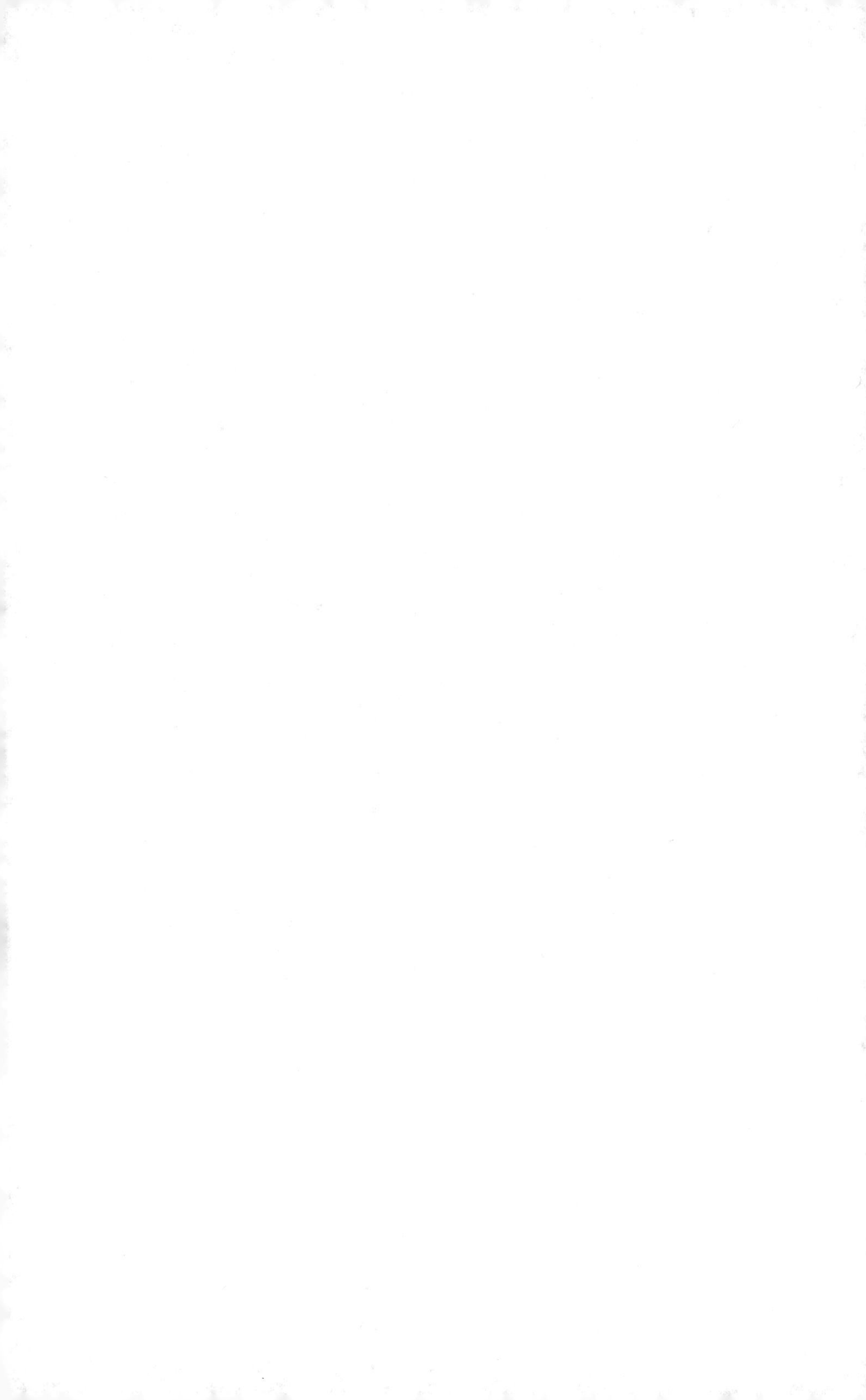

www.ingramcontent.com/pod-product-compliance
Lightning Source LLC
Chambersburg PA
CBHW071026250726
48653CB00005B/1730